GRANDMA RULES

T0040216

GRANDMA RULES

Notes on Grandmotherhood, the World's Best Job

Jill Milligan

with Michael Milligan

Illustrations by Adam Wallenta

Skyhorse Publishing

To the Special Grandmothers of Our Family
Alice "G.G.C." Cutler and Carolyn "Grandma Carol" Milligan
And Before Them
Ida "Buzzie" Cutler and Charlotte "Yayee" Milligan-Johnston
And to Grandmothers Everywhere

Skyhorse Publishing books may be purchased in bulk at special discounts for sales promotion,
corporate gifts, fund-raising, or educational purposes. Special editions can also be created to
specifications. For details, contact the Special Sales Department, Skyhorse Publishing, 307 West
36th Street, 11th Floor, New York, NY 10018 or info@skyhorsepublishing.com.

Skyhorse® and Skyhorse Publishing® are registered trademarks of Skyhorse Publishing, Inc.®,
a Delaware corporation.

Visit our website at www.skyhorsepublishing.com.

10 9 8 7 6 5 4 3 2 1

Paperback ISBN: 978-1-62873-773-8

Library of Congress Cataloging-in-Publication Data

Milligan, Jill.
Grandma rules : notes on grandmotherhood, the world's best job / Jill Milligan, with
Michael Milligan ; illustrations by Adam Wallenta.
p. cm.
ISBN 978-1-60239-683-8 (hardcover)
1. Grandmothers. 2. Grandparenting. 3. Milligan, Jill. I. Milligan,
Michael, 1947- II. Wallenta, Adam. III. Title.
HQ759.9.M54 2009
306.874'5--dc22
                              2009001213

Printed in China

CONTENTS

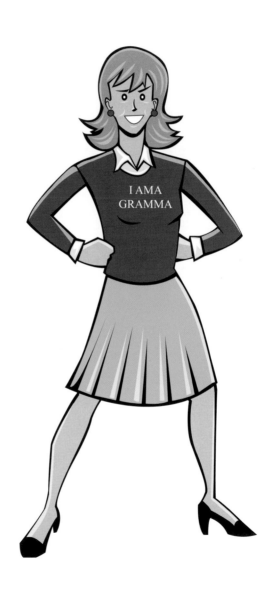

PREFACE

When I began writing this book, I spent the first four days staring at the same blank computer screen, wondering two things:

1. "How did I let myself get talked into this?"

And:

2. "Is 10 A.M. too early to hit the Chardonnay?"

There are some women who—no matter how they get themselves into a fix—will somehow find a way to blame their husbands. But thankfully, I am not one of those women. My husband is sweet, funny, loving, compassionate, and an amazing grandfather. He's all I've ever dreamed of . . . But then, I've had some weird dreams in my life.

But the more I think about it, this whole thing *is* kind of his fault. I mean, it all started about six months ago when his book, *Grandpa Rules*, was published. *Grandpa Rules* is Mike's funny account about becoming a grandfather, and its pages are full of anecdotes and advice to lovingly guide other baby boomer men as they shuffle their pasty-white legs down the path of Grandfatherhood. We were thrilled when *Grandpa* hit the bookstores. It began selling briskly; the reviews were positive; and best of all, our granddaughters thought it was way cool when they got to appear on a national television book interview with their "Buh-Buh." But in all the hoopla of Mike's book, something totally unexpected happened . . . A number of people suggested that I write "a funny book for grandmas."

That was very flattering; and I do, after all, have some qualifications. First and most importantly, I have over fourteen years' experience as the proud grandmother of four granddaughters: Sydni, Samantha, Alexandra, and Claire. The first three, ages fourteen, ten, and five are courtesy of my older daughter, Dionn, and her husband, Ron. Claire, two, was brought into the world by my daughter Mischon and her husband, Kevin. I can honestly say that all four of my wonderful granddaughters are genetically blessed with beauty, intelligence, wit, and good-heartedness. I can only assume that their occasional temper tantrums, their refusal to speak for days at a time, and their urge to wear brassieres at the age of six come from the other side of the family.

Second, I've done a fair amount of stand-up comedy at clubs in New York, Los Angeles and anywhere in between that would have me before the word got out.

So I felt okay about the experience and funny parts—but writing a book? What did I know about that? I decided to take advantage of being married to a writer and thought that I could learn a lot by watching him. Mike had started a new project, so I secretly observed him for a day to find out how a real writer works.

8:30 A.M.–10:00 A.M.: Read newspaper, drink coffee, use the bathroom, read the newspaper, have more coffee, and then use the bathroom again. (Note: Apparently there's a writer's rule that says no matter how many times you go into the bathroom, *do not* comb your hair.)

10:00 A.M.–11:30 A.M.: Go into the kids' old bedroom that became an office when they moved out, and sit at the computer wearing old boxer shorts you've slept in for the past three days. Top that off with a thirty-five year-old T-shirt from *The Jeffersons*, and you're good to go.

11:30 A.M.–11:31 A.M.: Make yourself presentable to go out in public.

11:31 A.M.–12:15 P.M.: To "get the creative juices flowing," drag the cobweb-covered bike from the garage for a brisk three-block ride to Starbucks. (Note: When the bike's rusty chain breaks at the 1½ block mark, you'll have to walk it the rest of the way.)

12:15 P.M.–1:30 P.M.: Drink skim lattes with fellow grandfathers and argue politics, make fun of young people (anyone under fifty), and debate where to find the best discount colonoscopies.

1:31 P.M.: Call wife to pick you up. Remind her to bring the SUV to haul home the broken bike.

1:45 P.M.: Arrive home. Go back into office, close the door, and play computer solitaire for two hours.

4:00 P.M.: Call it a day.

9:00 P.M.: Go to bed early to be fresh and raring to go when you get up at six the next morning.

To play golf.

I saw clearly that I was on my own, but I was not alone. Many of the grandmother advice, stories, and anecdotes you'll find in *Grandma Rules* come not only from me, but from my many grandmother friends as well. I hope that they'll bring smiles and chuckles to grandmothers of all ages, shapes, sizes, and levels of surgical enhancement. Some of you may be long-time grandmothers. Others might be—like me—a Baby Boomette, a member of the generation who's transitioned from hip huggers to hip replacement; from GTOs to HMOs, and from tie-dyed to "Who died?"

But regardless of your age or experience level, *Grandma Rules* is for all members and members-to-be of the wonderful sorority known as I Amma Gramma.

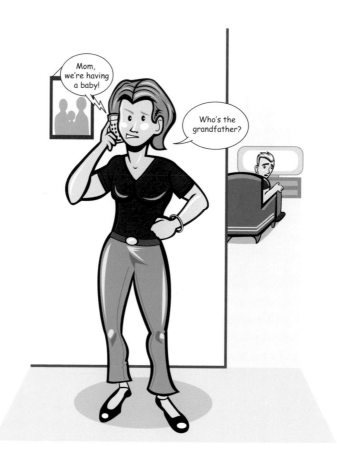

ONE

WHO ARE YOU CALLING "GRANDMA"?

*A*s a single mom of two teenage daughters, I was consumed with making sure they stayed on the straight and narrow. This became such an obsession that it stuck with me even after they were well into their twenties. That probably explains why, when my happily married twenty-five-year-old daughter called and said, "Mom, you're going to be a grandmother!" my knee-jerk response was, "Oh, great. Who's the grandfather?"

That was the first "grandma" joke I wrote for my act, and decided to introduce it into my routine at an appearance in front of my largest audience ever—a group of raucous senior citizens aboard a cruise ship.

The main ballroom was packed with over 350 people waiting anxiously to hear my act. Three hundred fifty people! I was so excited!

Until I found out I was the opening act for a bingo tournament.

But a gig's a gig, so I started by telling my audience how I'd been a young, suddenly single mother of two attractive and independent teenage daughters. And how—because "attractive" and "independent" can be a lethal combo for teenage girls—I was determined that they didn't become young, single mothers like I did. I insisted on meeting every boy my daughters dated. We discussed birth control, and

I even suggested that they might want to consider entering a convent. The fact they were Unitarians shouldn't be a deal breaker.

Okay, so Comedy Central never came calling, but those seniors enjoyed me enough that I was asked to perform again two days later . . . right before an ice sculpting demonstration.

Before I became a grandmother, I was—like most of you—a mother. So before getting into the grandmother years, I think it would be helpful to look at how the experience of motherhood affects that of grandmotherhood.

But first I'd like to talk about what every mother of a teenage daughter already knows: calling a teenage daughter "independent" is really just a euphemism for "devil child who cannot possibly be mine, and will somebody please come and take her away before she makes me crazy?"

If you say "Left," she says "Right." If you say "Hot," she says "Cold." If you say, "I don't want you going out with a guy with a nipple ring and tattoos," she says . . . well, I'll leave it to your imagination what she says.

The point is, I've often heard it said that "there's nothing like the bond between a mother and daughter." I've come to believe that to be so, but when those daughters were teenagers, that "bond" felt more like wearing a bra lined with porcupine quills.

During a few of these hair-pulling years, I worked with a woman named Mimi, who was also a single mom to two teenagers. But her warm, nurturing relationship with her children was the opposite of mine because of one important difference: While I was dealing with two daughters, Mimi was raising two teenage sons.

"They are so loving and responsible," she'd coo. "They make their own lunches, wash and iron their own clothes, and sometimes when I come home from work, they've got a delicious dinner waiting for me."

Whenever Mimi talked about what a wonderful relationship she had with her boys, I wondered how come it wasn't like that with my daughters and me. Their way of making their own lunches was lifting three bucks from my purse every morning to eat in the cafeteria. And the only thing they did with their laundry was toss it on the floor. And making me dinner? Only if you consider microwave popcorn fine dining. I was green with envy. Why didn't they do their own laundry or make me delicious meals like Mimi's sons did?

That's when I took a long, hard look at my parenting skills and arrived at a sobering conclusion: Mimi's sons were obviously gay. (Of course, I was just telling myself this to make myself feel better, and years later I learned that Mimi's older boy went on to play football in college, where he maintained a 1.8 GPA and impregnated an over-sexed, blonde Tri-Delt. But shucks, who hasn't?) Mimi's younger son, now thirty-three, is a surfer by day and by night pours drinks at a beach bar, where his work clothes consist of baggy shorts, faded T-shirts, and flip-flops. What self-respecting gay man would be caught dressing like that? That's about as likely as my husband walking out of the house for ten consecutive days with his pants properly zipped.

A few years after I met Mimi, I briefly dated a man who had custody of his teenage son. The boy seemed nice enough and was always pleasant and willing to engage in conversation. But with his father, I never heard the sixteen year-old say more than "yeah" and "no way, bro!" It wasn't like they didn't care for each other, because I could tell that they did. I guess fathers and sons just don't like talking about their feelings for each other . . . unless a son needs a loan document co-signed.

And finally, I once lived in the same condo complex as a single dad who'd been raising his sixteen year-old daughter since his wife passed away many years earlier. I don't know if it had anything to do with his daughter trying to fill in for her mother, but this striking girl was perfect. No spiked hair, no pierced nose, and no black mascara that made her look like Rocki Raccoon. She was polite, responsible, and had a relationship with her father that reminded me of Ryan and Tatum O'Neal. (Think *Paper Moon*, without the stints in rehab.)

So what was it with me and my teenage daughters being at each other's throats 24/7? Then, after thinking about all these different parent/child combinations, I had a revelation. If children, through no doing of their own, find themselves being raised by a single parent, it's best if they're raised by a parent of the opposite sex. Face it, dads don't get in catfights with daughters, nor do moms engage in shoe-throwing wars with sons.

If you doubt any of this, keep in mind that a coddled, young male child is sometimes referred to as a "Mama's Boy." Likewise, a daughter is often called "Daddy's Little Girl." But have you ever heard of a daughter called a "Mama's Little Girl?" Or a son being told to "Quit being such a Daddy's Boy?" Of course not, because neither of these would have any meaning or connotation; gender expectations are so very deep-rooted.

But that's for later. For now, I can tell you that my daughters and I survived the storm brought on by my single motherhood colliding with their teenage daughter-hood. Today, the three of us often laugh about the absurdity of those days, and I can happily report that both of my beautiful and talented daughters are college graduates, happily married, and very proud mothers.

Just like their mom.

To the guardian angel who's been looking out for us all these years, I want to offer a big "thank you" for all you've done. You have guided us through some rocky times and have helped us experience moments of great joy. And so far, one of the greatest joys was finding out I was going to be a grandmother.

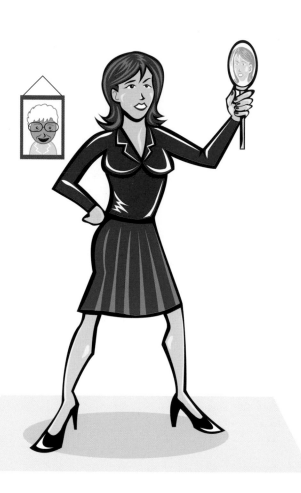

TWO

I GOT THE NEWS TODAY, OH BOY . . .

It was around dinnertime when my daughter and her husband called with the announcement that would enrich our lives from that day forward. I remember what time it was because when she put me on her speaker phone, I could hear my son-in-law clattering dishes in the background.

"Hi, Mom," Dee said. "How're you doing?

"Fine," I answered. "How're you?"

"Great," my son-in-law answered for them, as he bashed more dishes together. Then, for some odd reason, he added, "Hey, Jill. It's me, Ron." I wondered why he'd say that—who else would it be? Maybe with all the dish noise, he didn't want me to think Dee was having an affair with a busboy.

"We've got some news for you," Dee said coyly.

"You got your promotion?" I asked.

"No."

"Aw, don't tell me they gave it to that guy whose uncle works in Personnel . . ."

"Mom, they call it 'human resources' these days, and no, I'm still waiting to hear on the promotion."

"Okay," I said. "But if they give it to him, you can sue," I proclaimed with the legal certainty of one who never missed a single episode of *L.A. Law*.

"Mom, this is better than any promotion," Dee gushed. "See the thing is . . ."

But before she could finish, Ron could no longer contain his excitement and gleefully blurted: "We're pregnant!"

★   ★   ★   ★   ★

Time-out for a moment while I interrupt this heart-warming story to correct a misconception fathers-to-be seem to have.

Guys, it's wonderful and essential that you become part of the whole "having a baby" experience with your wives. But you need to remember this: *You are not—nor will you ever be—pregnant!*

A husband announcing, "Guess what? We're pregnant!" is like a wife announcing, "Guess what? We're having a vasectomy!"

Granted, you *are* the reason that the woman you love more than anyone in the world will soon become nauseous, grouchy, and in six short months will be able to buy her clothes at a sumo wrestler's garage sale.

And yes, you'll try to be patient and go out of your way to make her happy by rubbing her feet, running out to fulfill strange food requests at all hours, and insisting that she still looks beautiful even though she could have "Good-year" stenciled on her side.

But you are *not* pregnant. Because if *you* were pregnant and in *your* second trimester, you'd refuse to go to a party knowing you could only drink bottled water while your wife pounded back mojitos yelling, "Heck yeah, I'll have another one. *He's* driving!"

And if *you* were pregnant, would *you* be urging natural childbirth? Or, would you be demanding enough anesthesia to keep you happily sedated and pain-free until your new baby begins middle school?

So instead of "We're pregnant," I suggest you use "We're expecting," or "We're having a baby." If neither of these works for you, you can always use the goofy male standby of elbowing your buddy, pointing at your wife's stomach, and chuckling proudly as you stick out your chest like a rooster on parade.

Now back to my daughter's phone call . . .

★   ★   ★   ★   ★

The only thing I could say before I started crying was, "Ohmigod, Dee. Congratulations. I am so happy!" And I was. I couldn't believe it. My little baby was having a baby of her own. It was like no feeling I'd ever known.

My eyes were still misty an hour later when Mike got home from work. (I should tell you that he was producing a television show at the time, so his "work" consisted of sitting in a room with other grown men—all of whom resembled extras from *One Flew Over the Cuckoo's Nest*—and trying to make one another laugh. The only daily stress of his job seemed to be deciding which four-star restaurant they'd choose for lunch.)

When I turned to greet him, he could tell I'd been crying.

"What's wrong?"

"Dee called and . . ." I started choking up.

"That little suck-up with the uncle in Personnel got the promotion?! Dee's got more brains in her little finger than he's got in his whole butt-kissing body!"

"No," I said, smiling. "She's pregnant."

Mike was absolutely thrilled. He picked me up and whisked me like a teenager around the kitchen. "That's great news! Congratulations, Grandma!"

That's when time froze.

Grandma? I thought. Wow. Can he possibly be referring to me? And if so, how did this "grandma" thing happen? Where did the years go? I'd never thought of myself as old enough to be a Grandma. Oh, sure, I was thrilled at the prospect, but a small part of me was resisting. I was like an Ivory Soap Grandma—only *99.44* percent thrilled.

The remaining teensy-weensy 0.56 percent of the soon-to-be Grandma in me couldn't keep from flashing back forty years to when I was a six-year-old who pretended her ballet shoes were glass slippers. Seemingly overnight, I'd become a forty-six-year-old professional woman who was now worried about glass ceilings. And what happened to the fourteen-year-old Jill, a teeny-bopper who got weak-kneed over John, Paul, George, and Ringo? She's now an adult to whom John Paul was a pope, George was a president (twice), and Ringo was something that a lot of women like me said in our divorce settlements: "Oh, no, you don't, you snake! I'm not letting that ring go!"

I wondered how I went from a bouncy, happy-go-lucky teenager in a mini-skirt to a middle-aged mom in a mini-van, to a soon-to-be grandmother.

And finally, I thought back to the vivacious nineteen-year-old college student who took over the dance floor wearing a pair of tight, red, leather hot pants. Today, the only time my pants are hot is when I take them out of the dryer.

That's when I realized the reality of reaching grand-mother age might take some getting used to.

I thought back to my own grandmother—a kindly, white-haired woman named Buzzie—and wondered if I would seem as ancient to my grandchild as Buzzie seemed to me. I hoped not, because as a boomer grandma who grew up in the narcissistic "Think Young" generation, I was still very vain about such things as my boobs and my waistline.

Buzzie, on the other hand, was a rather round woman who didn't seem to care whether or not her boobs were even *above* her waistline.

When Mike finished whirling me and set me down, he must have noticed my faraway look.

"What's up?"

"Do I look old to you?" I asked.

"Old enough for what?" he answered with a grin.

"C'mon . . . Do you think I'm pretty?"

"Do you think I'm crazy? Of course I think you're pretty."

"You're just saying that," I said, hoping he wasn't just saying that.

"No, I'm not. In fact, I think you are beautiful."

"Really?"

"Absolutely." Then he put his arms around my waist—the waist that once looked so good in hip-huggers and a crop top. "In fact," Mike said, "I think you will be, without a doubt, one of the sexiest grandmas I've ever slept with!"

What a guy.

Then he announced that we needed to celebrate, and that I should pick any restaurant in the city for dinner. I chose my favorite place, a French bistro in Hollywood, not far from the studio where he worked. Even though it wasn't near our house, and he'd have to drive back to where he'd just come from, Mike never batted an eye.

"Excellent choice!" he said.

We had a perfectly delightful meal, where the main topic of discussion was grandparenthood and the excitement and challenges it would surely bring. It wasn't until dessert—when the maitre d' came to our table to chat—that I learned that Mike and all the writers had eaten lunch there that very day.

Mike just shrugged and smiled as the maitre d' moved off.

"Why didn't you say something?" I asked. "We didn't have to drive all the way back here."

"Of course we did," he said taking my hands. "If I'm taking the most beautiful grandmother on the planet out to dinner, it better be someplace special."

Like I said . . . What a guy.

I'll spare you the details, but when we got home I made sure that I was, without a doubt, the sexiest grandma he'd ever slept with.

And fourteen years and four beautiful, talented, loving, and perfect granddaughters later, I like to think that I still am.

Oh, and that 99.44 percent thing? It didn't take me long to get over that.

It vanished at the very moment I first held my two-minute-old granddaughter, Sydni.

Since then, I'm 100 percent pure Grandma.

THREE

GRANDMA 2.0

A CHILD'S BIRTHDAY CARD FOR GRANDMA (CIRCA 1958)

G is for the Gingham dresses you made my dolls.
R is for the Rhubarb pies you baked with care.
A is for the Aromas of cedar chests and old moth balls.
N is for the Nets you wore to cover your hair.
D is for the Dollars you sent every birthday.
M is for the Mah-jongg you loved to play.
A is for All the love I send to you this day.

AND NOW, THE 2014 VERSION

G is for the Gap, where you buy me tons of clothes.
R is for your Red ragtop Beemer with zebra seats.
A is for your Allergist, who stopped your runny nose.
N is for your Nutritionist, who took you off red meats.
D is for the Dermatologist who did your facial peel.
M is for Mud baths and how they make you feel.
A is because you're Awesome. And that's like, so totally for real!

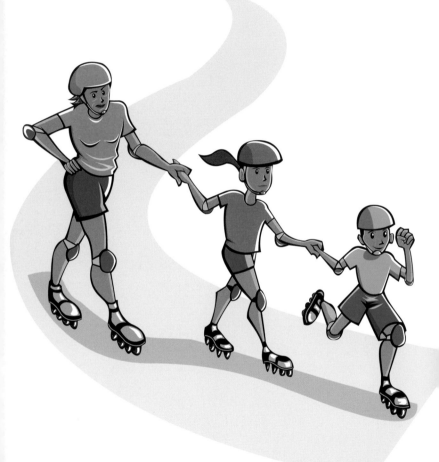

Obviously, there are huge differences between today's grandmothers and those of previous generations. We are younger, we are more active, and we are dedicated to the proposition that all men are created equal . . . unless we're married to him.

Today, the average age of a first-time grandmother is forty-seven, which indicates that we are becoming grand-mothers much younger than in previous generations. So it follows that we will likely be around for our grandchildren longer than our grandmothers were for us. Thus, if "seventy is the new fifty," then "*great*-grandmothers are the new grandmothers." I'm not sure what effect that will have on anything, but I suspect it won't be long before high school students everywhere will have a whole new generation to blame for not completing their homework assignments. "I woulda finished it, but, dude, my great-grandmother died."

The point is, today's grandmothers require a whole new set of tools and talents than those our grandmothers needed.

A: EXTRA LARGE SQUARE BAND-AIDS

Don't panic; these Band-Aids are not because your grand-child is likely to be injured under your watch.

No, the Band-Aids are for you.

You see, as a modern grandmother, don't you think it's finally time to cover up that tattoo you got way back during the Summer of Love? You know—the one with the psyche-delic dove flying toward the sun while carrying a peace sign in its mouth? The one you decided would look so totally groovy on the upper quadrant of your right breast? Well, thanks to the effects of time and gravity, what was once a gentle dove soaring toward the sun, now looks like an over-sized condor, nose-diving into a canyon of mashed potatoes.

So, unless you want that tattoo to embarrass your grandchild even more than it did your own daughter, cover it up.

For those of you who were forward-thinking enough to have your body art placed in a concealed location—say on your lower left buttock—you may not have to worry about covering that souvenir of your tequila-soaked spring break in Ft. Lauderdale. But only if you wear long pants. Because if you choose shorts, it's likely that over the past forty years, your purple tattoo of Jimi Hendrix has traveled south for the winter and is now living somewhere behind your left knee. Unless you want your tattoo to be mistaken for an ugly bruise, put a lid on it.

B: THUMB STRENGTH

"Do you think Grandma would buy some Girl Scout cookies?" I asked my mom during the first year of my brief Scouting career.

"I don't know," she said. "Why don't you write her a letter?"

"Couldn't I just call?" I asked. I didn't think hawking stale cookies merited a letter. Letters were for more important things like pen pals, or dumping a guy, or explaining to your cousin how you and her boyfriend got yourselves in that position during a game of Twister.

"Buzzie would enjoy a letter," Mom said. "Or don't you care about your grandmother enough to sit down and write one?"

What was it about parents of that generation that made them think that guilt would actually work on kids?

"Dear Buzzie," I wrote. "Hi, this is Jill. I joined the Girl Scouts because my mom thought it would teach me how to be responsible. I'm not sure how a dorky green dress and knee socks will do that, but I said I'd try it. We're having a cookie drive and if I don't sell twelve boxes, I can't go on our big outing to the Museum of Knot Tying. So would you like to buy a box or two? If not, that's okay, 'cause I already know how to tie a knot. Love, Jill. P.S. They're a dollar a box."

A week later, I got a letter back from my grandmother. I'm not sure how the mailman figured out where to deliver it, because I certainly couldn't read my grandmother's writing on the envelope. She was very old by this time, and her hands shook so much that she made Katharine Hepburn look like a diamond cutter. My mom couldn't make out Buzzie's message either, but the three crisp dollars in the envelope pretty much explained everything.

But alas, like many things of my childhood, letter-writing has gone the way of Flavor Straws, wax Halloween lips, and those matching outfits my parents brought home from Hawaii.

Today, we have text messaging—a communication method regularly used by more than 82 million people, 81,999,000 of whom are grandchildren. Studies show that the remaining 1,000 are "accidental texters" i.e., grandparents who push the wrong buttons while trying to dial 4-1-1 to find nearby restaurants that offer early bird dining.

Texting requires a great deal of speed and thumb strength, and since the most exerting thing your thumbs have done recently is turn the pages of the latest Janet Evanovich novel, you will need to develop the muscles in this digit if you want to communicate with your grandchildren.

Here are a few exercises you can do to help strengthen this important appendage.

1. See how long you can go with using only your thumbs to lift anything heavier than a cocktail weenie. If you

choose this method, be sure to have several aprons on hand, as well as a stockpile of Handi Wipes.

2. Recreate your odyssey of 1968 when you thumbed your way to San Francisco. But this time, you'll have better luck since you are no longer making your "no shaving my legs" statement. Also, remember to accept no rides from chatty Hare Krishnas.

3. If you decide against the first two, you can practice unsnapping your bra with one hand, then with the other. Then, after you've mastered this maneuver, strive for the impossible by trying to teach it to your husband or boyfriend.

After you add muscle tone to your great evolutionary gift of opposing thumbs, you will use them as your primary tools when you communicate with your grandkids through TMS. TMS stands for Text Message Shorthand, which uses more acronyms and abbreviations than Dow Jones. For example, would you know how to respond if you received this message from Carrie, your college freshman grand-daughter? "HI, GM. HIG? IN PS 4 SPR BK. CU MON. HAND. 459, C."

Because you've done your TMS homework, you know that "HI, GM. HIG?" translates to "Hi, Grandma, How's it going?" And that "IN PS 4 SPR BK" represents "I'm in Palm Springs for spring break." "CU MON" is undoubt-edly "See you Monday;" "HAND" is "Have a nice day." And surely you'd know that "459" means "I love you," because the letters "I," "L," and "Y" are on the numbers 4,5, and 9 of the cell phone's keypad.

Of course you would.

Then, to show your granddaughter that you're a lot hip-per than her other grandmas, you should respond to her as follows: "HC! (Hi, Carrie) AGH (All good here.) MOOD. (Munching Out On Dinner.) HV FN, BBG! (Have Fun, But Be Good!) MS U. (Miss You) C4N, (Ciao for now) G. (Grandma)."

Or if you wanted to give up and go old school, you could call her back.

C: FREQUENT FLYER MILES

Even if your grandchildren live only a short plane trip away, and you think you have plenty of air miles banked for every occasion, listen to what I am about to tell you: You are wrong. You can *never* have enough miles. Why? Because your grandchild's other grandmother lives only three blocks away and babysits twice a week, and at this very moment is probably telling him that his other grandma—the one who practically lives in a foreign country and, at her age, still goes to Rolling Stones concerts—is probably just too busy to see him.

So pull out that gold card and rack up those miles! And when your husband sees the monthly bill and nearly explodes, just explain that all those charges are for presents for the grandkids. Odds are, he will smile and congratulate you for keeping on top of things.

D: A GYM MEMBERSHIP

A few years ago, when my young granddaughters were try-ing maneuver their way through the FEMA disaster area known as my garage, they spied my skis. This discovery was soon followed by the unearthing of my rollerblades.

"Cool!" they said. "Whose are these?" they wanted to know.

"Mine," I told them.

"No. Really," the youngest insisted, reacting as though I'd just told her I'd recently had lunch with the tooth fairy *and* Dora the Explorer. At first, I didn't understand their surprise; I grew up on the slopes of the Sierras, and I'd been skiing since I was six. And over the years, rollerblading has not only kept me in skiing shape, but has also given me the opportunity to require the services of some very cute emergency room doctors. Why were my granddaughters so surprised that I'd be doing such things?

Then I thought back to my grandmother again and tried to imagine her skiing or rollerblading. No way; in fact, I'm fairly certain that she didn't even know how to ride a bike. Once, however, I did see her smiling as she rode down an escalator.

With my skeptical granddaughters looking on, I strapped on my in-line skates and took off. I hadn't roller bladed in several years, so I was a little wobbly at first. But after awhile I picked up some speed and was soon zooming down the sidewalk at nearly 2 mph! I was soon exhausted and wanted to quit, but with the girls cheering me on, I kept at it for nearly 30 minutes, all without a fall.

When their parents arrived a few hours later to pick them up, my granddaughters couldn't wait to tell them what they'd seen.

"Guess what, Mom!" Sydni screeched to my daughter. "Gaji knows how to rollerblade!" ("Gaji" is what my granddaughters call me. More on that later.)

"And she can ski, too!" said Samantha.

"I know," my daughter told her. "That's where I learned."

"She's going to take us this winter," Syd chirped to my son-in-law. "She wants to teach us, too!"

A few days later, I learned that on their drive home, they made all the plans for a January ski trip. But while they were in their car, booking condos on their cell phones, I was in pain on our sofa, trying to figure out how thirty minutes of rollerblading made my thighs feel like they'd been given acupuncture with hot fireplace pokers.

I had signed up a gym for three years earlier, and the next morning I called and booked a few sessions with a fitness counselor. Then, before I hung up, I made sure to find out where the gym was located.

A few days later, once my legs were operating again, I had my first session with my Fitness Adonis . . . er, counselor. In his mid-twenties, Eric had long black hair and a body more chiseled than the Ten Commandments.

"So, Jill," he said, studying the form I'd filled out. "You're here because . . . ?"

Because you're a heck of a lot cuter than my Thigh-Master, is what I was thinking.

But "I just want to get into a little better shape," is what I said. Eric nodded, and then he began looking me over to see how much work I needed, and how much he could actually accomplish.

As he made notes on my body, he reminded me of the auto shop guy who checked out my car when I took it in for some body work a few weeks earlier.

And like the auto guy, I could tell Eric was thinking, "A little ding here, a little dent there, but overall, it's in pretty good shape. By the way, nice headlights."

When the auto shop guy finished his inspection, he asked me how old the car was and when I told him, he was quite surprised. "Really? Doesn't look it. You must take good care of it."

"I try," I told the car guy. "My husband helps."

I suspected that Eric would be equally amazed when I told him that I was old enough to be a grandmother. He'd probably be so stunned that he'd faint dead away and land smack dab on his amazingly tight glutes.

"You see," I said to Eric, "I promised to take my grand-kids skiing."

"You're a grandmother?" he asked, doing a real good job of hiding his surprise. Figures . . . He must be another out-of-work, wannabe actor.

"That's right. Seven years now," I boasted.

"Wow!" he said. So he *was* surprised. But before I could break into a girlish grin, he continued. "We just started a workout program that would be perfect for you," he said. "It's just for seniors, and we're calling it Silver Sneakers."

Judging from his pride, I guessed that he thought up that name all by himself.

I never saw Eric again after that. I decided that I'd get into shape on my own, because my sneakers were nowhere close to being silver.

Three months later, I was skiing at Heavenly Valley with my granddaughters. They're good athletes, and after two days with me, they were safely skiing down intermediate slopes with absolutely no problem.

"Okay, girls, the hill's about to close," I told them as I started off toward the lodge.

"Just one more run, Gaji! Please?"

Even though my thighs were tingling after a day of non-stop skiing, how could I say "No" to those beautiful faces?

So we hopped on a chair lift and off we went. Halfway down our last run of the day, my granddaughters spied a trail they hadn't skied on yet.

"Can we go this way?" they begged.

I checked the trail map and saw that they could easily handle it. "Sure," I said, telling them to go first and I'd follow in case they needed help.

As they took off, I noticed the trail sign and smiled, thinking of my grandmother Buzzie.

The trail my granddaughters had chosen was named "Escalator Down."

And as they slalomed down the slope, I realized that I was about their age when Buzzie had patiently taught me to knit. And even though my first and only knitting project was a misshapen, scrawny coaster that was too puny to accommodate anything much larger than a shot glass, my grandmother was thrilled that she had taught me something. Just like I was thrilled at teaching my granddaughters how to ski. And as I took off after them, nothing could have made me more proud, nor my quads more sore. Maybe next time, I'll teach them to knit.

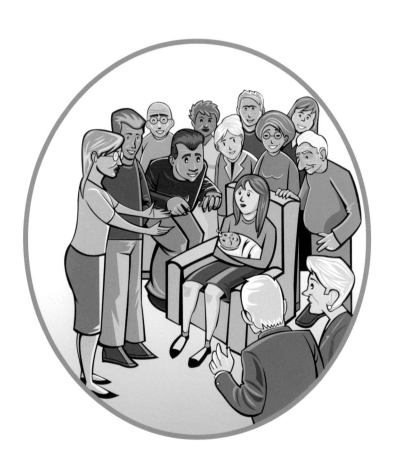

FOUR

TWO, FOUR, SIX, EIGHT, WHO DO WE APPRECIATE?

Sean, a handsome, twenty-five-year-old Irishman walked into a bar in Manhattan and explained to the bartender that he'd just been transferred to New York from Ireland. Sean had rented a nearby apartment, and this bar reminded him of his pub back home. They chatted for awhile longer, then Sean ordered three pints of Guinness.

"Sure," said the barkeep. "Are you expecting friends?"

"Oh, no," said Sean. "I've not yet had the opportunity to make friends in New York. But I miss my two lovely grandmothers in Ireland very much. You see, my parents died when I was just a wee lad, and both my grandmums raised me. I'd like to have a pint with each of them," he said.

The bartender was touched by his sentiment and set three pints on the bar in front of Sean.

Sean hoisted the pint on his right and said, "To my beautiful granny in Dublin. I love you more than life itself." Then he slowly emptied the glass.

Then he hoisted the pint on his left. "To my saintly grandmum in Galway. Though we are miles apart, may our hearts always be together."

And then he slowly drank the second pint down.

And last, he took the pint in the middle and knocked it back. Then, without a word, he dabbed his eyes, paid his tab, and left.

Every night, Sean came in and drank one pint for his grandmother in Dublin, one for his grandmother in Galway, and one for himself. It was always the same.

So moved was the bartender by this young man's devotion to his grandmothers that he told a few other patrons about it, and soon people from other neighborhoods would come in to see this fine young man honor his grandmothers.

This went on every single night for over ten months.

Then one evening, with the bar packed, Sean walked in and the bartender began filling three glasses, but Sean stopped him.

"Only two glasses tonight, please," Sean said soberly.

A hush fell over the crowd. "My gosh, Sean," the bartender said, fighting back tears. "Did something happen to your grandmother in Dublin?"

"No," Sean said. "She's fine, thank you."

"Oh, no . . ." said the barkeep. "So it was your grandmum in Galway."

"Not at all. She's fit as a fiddle."

The bartender was stumped. "So why only two pints?"

"Oh, that's because of me," said Sean. "I quit drinking for Lent."

★   ★   ★   ★   ★

Like Sean and kids who grew up in the fifties, I only had two grandmas and two grandpas, although I never met my grandfathers because they died well before my grandmothers did. Unfortunately for men, this trend continues today, and women live, on average, two years longer than men. I'm not sure exactly why this is, but I have a theory that as men get older, they are penalized one heartbeat for every time they argue with the television, refuse to obey maps, or call their wives "the old ball and chain."

Statistics from the 2000 U.S. Census indicate that the boomer population—meaning anyone born between 1946 and 1964—consists of almost 83 million people, which represents 36% of the people in the U.S. today. After factoring in that this population is 51% female, we see that a high percentage of women are between the age of 44 and 62. I think this suggests three things:

1) There will be more grandmothers today than ever before
2) Many of today's grandchildren will have *at least* two grandmothers
3) There will be no government bail outs necessary for anyone involved in the hip replacement business

But because of today's increased divorce rate, modern grandkids will likely have more grandparents that we did. If you ask my granddaughters how many grandmothers and grandfathers they have, they'll no doubt answer "six."

Oh, I know what a lot of you are thinking . . . "Oh, sure, but a grandchild really only has two *real* sets of grandparents." Oh yeah? Well, try explaining that to the grandchildren.

Let me tell you about my family, which is not all that different from lot of American families—unless you count my Uncle Linus, who is now living in Brazil as my Aunt Lynn.

My first husband and I were married in the sixties when we were still in college. We stayed married for seven years, during which time we created our two exquisite daughters, who are now forty and thirty-six.

Following our divorce, I'd be lying if I claimed that my ex and I were friendly. In fact, I'm always enormously skeptical when I hear it said (usually by a woman), "Oh, yes, Bill and I are divorced. But he's still my best friend." Who is she kidding? If he was her best friend, why did they get divorced? What? He never put the cap back on the toothpaste? He insisted on having curtains made out of Schlitz Pop Tops? He made fun of her Ricky Nelson records?

If your ex is your best friend, I suggest you hurry out to happy hour at the Ramada and make some new friends, or perhaps you should join a dating service. Or, if you're more of a masochist and would like a friend who loves you one day, but rejects and ignores you the next, get a cat.

A few years after our divorce, my ex-husband and I had moved on, and he married a very nice and vivacious woman with whom he will soon celebrate his 25th wedding anniversary. I, on the other hand, had my hands full working and raising the girls. I wasn't particularly looking for a relationship.

Then I met the man I've been with for the past sixteen years and plan on being with for the next sixty.

And the meeting was all quite accidental. At least that's what he thought.

In the late eighties, I was in the corporate travel business, and spent a lot of time on airplanes traveling within California and Nevada. Early one morning, I was waiting to board a commuter flight from Los Angeles to Reno and as usual, nearly all of the passengers were exactly like me—professional worker bees on their way to, or coming home from, some sort of business meeting. All the women wore pressed skirts and jackets, and the men were in dark business suits . . . except for a guy with long shaggy hair who was hurrying to the boarding podium, trying to deal with a carry-on bag and a Styrofoam cup of steaming coffee.

He was decked out in faded jeans, a Hawaiian shirt, baseball cap, flip-flops, and looking more Marx Brothers than Brooks Brothers. He'd apparently overslept, as it appeared that he'd thrown on his clothes just in time to make his flight. My trained eye told me that this guy was about my age and definitely *not* a business traveler . . . unless his business was something like bead-stringing. Or bong manufacturing.

I can't remember exactly what he said to the gate attendant, but I do remember it being very funny. Then, after receiving his boarding pass, he headed for a chair and spilled a good amount of his hot coffee on his bare toes as he walked past me.

"Agh!" he said to no one in particular. Then he looked to me. "Did I get any on you?" he asked.

"No," I answered.

"Good," he said, relieved. "At four bucks a pop, I shouldn't be throwing this stuff around." Then he hopped over to a seat to wait for boarding.

One of the perks of working in the travel business is receiving upgrades, and I'd snagged the very last first-class seat. If I had to be on yet another airplane, at least I'd have enough legroom and a free mimosa. So why was I walking up to the gate attendant about getting my seat changed? "Where's *he* sitting?" I whispered, indicating Mr. Flip-Flops.

She checked her computer. "17-C," she told me.

"Anything open next to him?" I asked hopefully.

"17-B," she said. "Why?"

Why? I wanted to tell her that when you travel a lot, flying becomes a real bore. You've read all the in-flight magazines cover to cover, airplane coffee begins to taste like something that came out of a goat, and any conversation you might have with a fellow passenger usually devolves into discussing your companies, your health plans, and your uninteresting jobs. I had a feeling talking to this guy might make the flight seem much shorter. "Great," I said, handing over my first-class ticket for a cramped middle seat in coach. "17-B it is."

It was as easy as that; the only hard part was my trying to act surprised when we "happened" to be sitting next to each other.

★ ★ ★ ★ ★

We had a most enjoyable flight and some good laughs. I told him I going to Reno for a sales meeting; he was headed there to watch his teenage son's baseball team from L.A. play in a tournament.

"You got kids?" he asked.

We soon discovered that my two daughters were practically the same ages as his two sons. But before you start thinking this meeting is headed toward a Brady Bunch moment, put away your Kleenex. We arrived in Reno after a one-hour flight, got off the plane, thanked each other for the conversation, shook hands, and that was that.

But That wasn't even close to That.

Because Fate apparently had other plans for us.

You see, I was ticketed to return to Los Angeles Sunday evening, but my mom lived in Reno and talked me into having dinner and spending the night. So I booked a 6:15 flight for Monday morning.

And guess who happened to be on the very same flight? And wearing the same Hawaiian shirt!

Of course, we sat together again and swapped stories of our Reno visits. When I mentioned that I had an interest in comedy, Don Ho-Ho-Ho said that he knew some "comedy people" in L.A. and would be happy to introduce me to them. *He knows comedy people?* I thought. *What does this guy do?*

"Oh, I'm a writer," he said, mildly.

"Really?" I said. "And what do you write?"

He explained that he was a writer and producer for a comedy show at Paramount called *Dear John*, and asked if I'd heard of it.

Of course I'd heard of it. "You're a comedy writer for television?" My voice must have contained some skepticism, because he answered with:

"What did you expect—a joy buzzer and a squirting flower?" Then he offered that if I'd ever like to see the show filmed, I should call the number he was scribbling on a napkin they'd given him with his coffee. He apologized for not having a business card, but he thought they were pretentious.

When we deplaned in Los Angeles Mike said, "Nice meeting you, Jill. Again."

"Same here," I told him.

As I walked toward the parking shuttles, and he in the opposite direction to a line of taxis, I made a note to be sure to call him as soon as I could.

★　★　★　★　★

And it only took me a year.

He later told me that when his assistant buzzed into his office, saying "There's a Jill calling for you. She said she met you on an airplane?" he remembered me immediately.

So I guess I made a good impression.

I'll cut to the chase here. I took him up on his offer to see a filming of *Dear John*, and Mike was very gracious, making sure that everyone met "his friend, Jill." And that's what we were—friends. But what I didn't know was that Mike's marriage was, sadly, unraveling, and well . . . yadda-yadda-yadda. The point is, a few years later he found himself divorced and at a candlelight dinner with me.

And that fire has not dimmed since.

This long tour of my family tree house is only meant to give you a glimpse into how we—and many families like ours—have been brought together into one, big, happy brood simply by one spectacular occurrence: the arrival of our first grandchild.

True, our family may contain more grandparents than a St. Mary's bingo game, but we truly enjoy the arrangement.

And we like to think our grandkids enjoy it, too.

Not long ago, our granddaughter Samantha was in a school play in which she had a part as one of many singing trees in a forest. A week before her stage debut, she called to make sure we'd be there.

"Of course we will," I told her, explaining that we'd be making the five-hour drive so we'd arrive in plenty of time.

"Oh, good," she said with excitement. "I told my friend Jasmine that all *six* of my grandparents were coming!" she chirped. Then she added, "Jasmine said, 'You have six grandparents? I only have two. You are like, so totally lucky!'"

And all of her grandparents couldn't agree more.

FIVE

MOTHER OF THE MOTHER, OR MOTHER OF THE DAD, ONE WAY OR THE OTHER, NONE OF IT'S BAD

As most new grandmothers learn very early on—sometimes painfully—there is a distinct difference between being the mother of a new mother versus being the mother of a new father.

Let's say your daughter-in-law, Felicia, is about to give birth to your first grandchild. Felicia's husband—who is your son—is a fine young man, and a tender, loving husband. You are a world-renowned OB-GYN *and* pediatrician, and you regularly lecture at the world's finest universities on the subject of new mothers and child care. You are also a former fashion model who, even at fifty-two, is still frequently mistaken for Christie Brinkley. You are totally gaga over your husband of thirty years, the handsome and athletic CEO of a non-profit that's dedicated to finding a cure for disease, world hunger, and paper cuts. Your daughter-in-law Felicia loves and admires you for so many reasons, not the least of which is because you saved her life at her engagement party when she began choking on a wedge of overcooked tofu.

You are the ideal person for any anxious first-time mother to have with her during delivery.

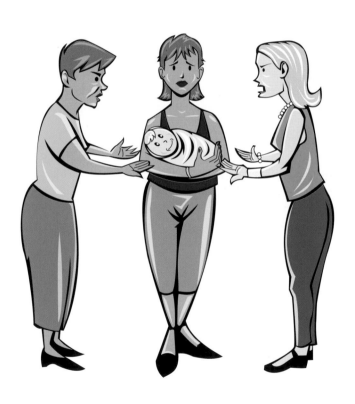

Felicia's mother, Viola, is a part-time palm reader with three failed marriages under her expansive belt. She currently lives with her latest boyfriend, a fifty-five-year-old professional dog walker, whom she met in a support group for people who are addicted to Spiro Agnew memorabilia.

So the choice is clear. When Felicia gives birth, who will she want at her side?

Hint: Not you.

That's right. Even though Felicia adores you, and tells everyone that you are the most fantastic mother-in-law in the world, the "in-law" part still only gets you a silver medal. But you shouldn't feel the least bit slighted, because the reality is that most new mommies want their own mommy at their side for the first week or so.

A respected physician we know attributes this to a phenomenon he calls the T.U.C.—Trans-Uterine Connection. Our doctor friend has read many technical papers that explore inherited DNA tendencies, tissue amalgamation as it pertains to the female reproductive system, and the reliability of inner-birth canal, trans-generational genetic identification. Unfortunately, none of these have even a scintilla of relevance to his theory of T.U.C., which he hit upon during a discussion with six other grandfathers in his poker group. Basically, the men who were fathers of daughters told how their wives were in the delivery room for every scream. The fathers of sons said their wives only got a call once the birth was over.

"Would you like me to come right away?" each mother asked of her son.

"Nah, that's okay, Mom. Jenny's mom is here."

But you should take heart in knowing that once your daughter-in-law and your new grandchild have been sufficiently pampered and loved by the "other" grandmother, you are absolutely free to spoil away.

For grandmothers who have daughters, I'm sure you've experienced T.U.C. firsthand.

But for the mothers of sons, many of whom will have their feathers temporarily ruffled, be assured that your grandchild will be unaffected by this phenomenon, and will love both grandmothers equally. And fear not; mothers of sons are imposed upon to babysit just as frequently as the T.U.C. grandmother.

There is, however, an important warning for Mothers of Daughters: Remember that the shelf life of T.U.C. is about two weeks. Just because your daughter wanted you when her baby was born and immediately afterward don't think that she will want or seek your advice as the child grows.

It does not give you carte blanche to say things to your daughter like, "That's not how you breast feed! Let me show you how I did it with you." Or, as the child gets older, the T.U.C. does not entitle you to make fun of contemporary parenting concepts and terminology.

For example, when you hear your daughter give your young grandson a "time-out" for misbehaving, you should refrain from saying, "*Time-out*? What is he, a two-year-old or a hockey player?" And if you should hear that your granddaughter is off on a "play date," bite your tongue instead of blurting, "*Play date*? She has to make a date to go play? What do you call eating lunch around here . . . a meal date?"

Another new trend going on today is the formation of "mommy groups," a modern networking system in which mothers of toddlers get together and discuss current child-raising issues. Today's "mommy groups," many of which have their own websites and charge monthly membership dues, are a lot more structured than when I was a young mother. Our "mommy groups," were called "Hey, why doesn't everybody come over for dinner? And bring the kids!" groups. Our children would get to know each other by playing, and the only expense was the cost of a few jugs of Annie Green Springs and a crock pot of sloppy joes. That seemed to work okay for us.

But recently, I learned of a trend that's becoming more and more popular within these mommy groups. And this one is so deliciously bizarre that no grandmother worth her AARP card should be expected to hold her tongue when she hears it:

Business cards for two-year-olds.

That's right. "Business" cards that list the child's name, contact information, availability for play dates, likes, dislikes, nap schedule, and food preferences, etc. Moms create these cards for their toddlers and then pass them out to other moms, hoping to find "like-minded" playmates. Like-minded? At two years old?

If this wacky trend catches on, will it be long before there's a website for toddlers to find their soulmates? Imagine . . .

- Name: Edgar Winterhalter, Jr.
- Age: 25 (months)
- Contact: edgar@over-the-top-mom.com
- Availability: See Playdate Calendar on website. But hurry; bookings going faster than my grandpa's hair.
- Likes: Baby Einstein videos (especially the one about atom-splitting), Raffi CD's.
- Dislikes: Uncle Steve and the word "no!"
- Favorite Food: organic eggplant and tofu rolls with molé.

- Seeking: Single, like-minded male or female for going down slides, playing in sandboxes, and removing diapers in public. Those with teething issues need not respond.

So far, I think this business card phenomenon is limited to small pockets of the Golden State. Let's hope it dies out before it spreads across the country like other unfortunate trends that gained footing here in California.

We already feel bad enough about the word "dude," Richard Nixon, and Taco Bell.

SIX

GRANDMA "X," GRANDPA "Y"

*W*hen Alice, a sixty-five-year-old grandmother, arrived to babysit her four-year-old grandson, she was holding a brightly wrapped package.

"Come see what your Gramma Alice bought you!" she said to her grandson. The little guy tore open the package and pulled out an outfit of matching shorts, shirt, and hat.

"Mom, that's sweet," said her daughter. "But you didn't have to do that."

"He'll look adorable in it," Alice said, dressing her grandson in his new outfit of matching shorts, shirt, and hat. "You can wear this when Nana takes you to the beach today."

"Mom, no beach today," said her daughter. "There's a high surf warning."

"Who's surfing?" Alice asked. "We'll just walk along the water and . . ."

"Mom, please, no beach."

"But . . ."

"Mother!" Alice's daughter said, losing her patience. "I don't want you taking him to the beach today. Understand?"

Alice sighed and gave in. "Okay, no beach . . ."

Then Alice's daughter kissed them both and left for an appointment, saying she'd be back at four.

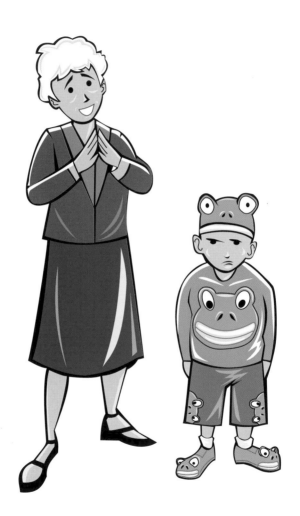

"What a shame," said Alice, looking at her grandson in his matching shorts, shirt, and hat. "You look just scrumptious."

"Beetz!" the little guy begged. "I wanna go beetz!" he continued.

He looked so cute in his new outfit.

"Surf, schmurf," Alice said as she took her grandson by the hand and headed out the door. They'd only stay an hour; that would be plenty of time for Alice to show off her grandson in his new outfit.

Just as her daughter said, the waves were very big, so they walked a safe distance from the water.

Then, without any warning, an enormous wave engulfed the shore, knocking her over and taking her grandson out to sea. By the time Alice got to her feet, all she could see was his head bobbing in the distance.

"Oh God," she pleaded to the heavens. "Please, God. If you bring my grandson back, I'll never ask you for anything again. Nothing! I promise!"

Suddenly, another huge wave crashed onto the shore and sure enough, it gently deposited her grandson onto the sand, completely unharmed, but now only wearing his matching shorts and shirt. She looked heavenward once more. "What? No hat?"

★   ★   ★   ★   ★

It's no secret that grandmothers love shopping for their grandkids, and there are several reasons for this. First, we enjoy spoiling them. Second, we want them look nice. And third, we want their other grandmas see what good taste we have.

But I've noticed that most grand*fathers*, wearing their Y chromosome like a badge of honor, generally have absolutely no interest in shopping for their grandchildren.

In fact, let's see how Alice's story would have gone if there were a grandpa involved . . .

★ ★ ★ ★ ★

Alice's husband Leon was driving them to their daughter's house to babysit their four-year-old grandson on a summer afternoon. Stopped at a red signal, Leon cursed the delay and blamed the mayor, the planning commission, and the Victoria's Secret billboard for causing so much more traffic than there was when he retired here ten years ago.

Ignoring him from the passenger seat, Alice noticed a beach outfit in the window of a children's store on the corner. It would look absolutely perfect on their grandson.

"Leon, pull over," she said with some urgency.

"I can't just 'pull over,'" he said.

"Why not? You're in the right lane."

"Of course I am," said Leon with purpose, knowing full well that making a left turn at this signal was the shorter route to his daughter's house. But since reading in his AARP magazine about how much time is wasted waiting to turn left, Leon now plans his itineraries so that he makes right turns only.

Before Alice could say another word, the light turned green and Leon sped off on his more circuitous route to their daughter's place.

When they arrived, their daughter could tell they'd been arguing.

"I saw the cutest beach outfit for Dusty," Alice explained. "But Parnelli Jones here wouldn't stop."

"Aw, the kid's already got more outfits than Liberace," Leon said. Then he turned to his grandson and pulled out a crisp twenty dollar bill. "Besides, Dusty, what would you rather have: a new outfit that would look better on a girl, or a trip to the ice cream store with LaLo?"

"Eyeth queam!" shouted the toddler.

"See you later, ladies," Leon said with a victorious smile. Then he took his grandson's hand and the two of them left for Ben and Jerry's, which was only three blocks—and five right turns—away.

★　★　★　★　★

Grandmothers and grandfathers each have their favorite spots to shop for their grandkids. Grandmothers go to malls. Grandfathers go to ATMs.

But an affection for shopping is certainly not the only area in which males and females vary. Here are just a few of the differences between grandmothers and grandfathers. . . .

THE AGING PROCESS

First of all, getting old is not a "process." Making Velveeta is a process. Turning cucumbers into pickles is a process. Trying to fully understand Liza Minnelli's marriages is a process. For women, aging is a curse. And not the kind that lasts only five days a month.

And while women will do everything in their power to stave it off, men actually seem to accept it. If you doubt this, take an inventory of the products *you* have in your bathroom cabinet: Three crowded shelves of moisturizing creams, hydrating beauty fluids, wrinkle balms, rejuvenators, skin toners . . . Then look in your husband's bathroom cabinet: Right Guard, a nail clipper, Cruex, and what's left of the Musk Oil he bought the night he took you to the Bee Gees concert.

At even the slightest trace of a facial blemish, women get facials, mud wraps, and exfoliating treatments.

Men grow a beard.

I spoke to a prominent plastic surgeon here in Los Angeles, and he told me that 97 percent of his elective facial cosmetic surgery patients are women. And of the 3 percent of his male patients, most are under the age of thirty-five. So I'm guessing that his few male patients who have plastic surgery and are over thirty-five fall into two groups: a) older actors, or b) Bruce Jenner.

And if a grandmother discovers that she has some unwanted flab on her rear or stomach, she can choose liposuction.

Men choose Sansabelt.

Which brings us to . . .

CLOTHING

Because today's grandmothers are younger than previous generations, the old idea of "grandma clothes" has gone the way of calf-length floral dresses, black leather "nun" shoes, and knee-high hosiery. If my grandmother wanted something stylish, she'd pull out her Singer. Today's grandmothers pull out our gold cards. The only line between clothes for younger women and those of us who are older is a hemline.

Today's grandfathers, however, don't seem to be the least bit concerned about style and have somehow gotten it into their Rogained heads that the most important clothing consideration is that of comfort. This explains why it's not uncommon to see a grandmother in brightly colored, stylish, above-the-knee dress having an early-bird dinner with her husband, who's wearing a pair of frayed khakis he's had since the Carter administration, and his "new" shirt, a spiffy button-down that he got for a buck at the thrift shop.

Perhaps because men know that they don't live as long as we do is why they spend so little time selecting clothes when they get dressed. That's the only explanation I have for what happened at my house just last week.

Our friends were picking us up at 7 o'clock for a dinner out, followed by a visit to a jazz club. It was 6:45; I'd been trying on outfits since 5:30, and our California King bed was blanketed with my rejects. Mike, on the other hand, just got home from golf and was having a martini in his underwear while he watched SportsCenter in the den. I yelled at him to hurry up as I checked myself in the mirror and decided that the pants/sweater combo I finally chose was completely wrong.

Five minutes before our friends were due to arrive, I came to the conclusion that I had absolutely *nothing* to wear. I heard Mike get out of the shower and spray on deodorant; and even though I was once again down to panties and bra, I urged him hurry up so he didn't make us late, figuring offense is always the best defense.

"Have you seen my khakis?" he called to me.

"They're in the dirty clothes," I answered.

"Why?"

"Because they were dirty," I lied about his most comfortable pants. The truth was, they were clean, but at their age, who could tell?

Five minutes later, our doorbell rang. "Can you get that?" I called, buttoning the 24th blouse I'd tried on in the past forty-five minutes.

"No prob," he answered. "But hurry up, okay?" He took all of five minutes to get ready.

Ten minutes later, I came out of the bedroom, finally ready to go. Our friends, Augie and Jean, were sitting with Mike in the living room, sipping wine. Jean had obviously spent as much time as I did getting ready, and looked terrific. Augie and Mike, on the other hand, looked like two-thirds of the Kingston Trio: they were both wearing old, worn khakis (Mike's were wrinkled from being in the hamper), long-sleeved oxford shirts, and beat-up loafers.

The guys must have planned it this way, knowing that if either Jean or I criticized our husband's outfit, we'd be criticizing the other guy's clothes as well.

Sometimes, it's better to shut up and smile.

"Well, let's go," Mike said, putting his arm around me. "Dang, we're a handsome group," he said as we left.

I resented that. How dare he lump me and Jean—who'd both spent hours getting ready—with him and Augie, who looked like they dressed in a tornado?

Finally, if you still think that dressing for comfort isn't important to your grandpa-husband, try this little test to beat him at his own game:

The two of you are going to a 5:30 movie; it's 5:00, and he's ready to go—wearing old sweat pants, a tee-shirt from his college fraternity and a pair of sneakers he got at a garage sale. As you sit on the sofa reading, he checks his watch nervously. He doesn't want to be late because even though the theater is only three blocks away, he has this new system about making right turns only.

"Aren't you gonna get ready?" he asks.

"In a minute," you say, just like he always does. "It won't take me long."

"Right . . ." he mumbles under his breath.

At 5:10, get off the sofa and go in to change. (*Note: Here's the important part.*)

1. Put on something even more raggedy than what he's wearing. (I know it's unlikely that you own anything that awful, but do your best.)
2. Go into the bathroom and *wash off* all your makeup.

3. Once that's done, hurry to the kitchen and spray your hair with PAM to give it a lived-in "comfortable" look, just like his.

4. Put on the sneakers you use exclusively for painting and tile grouting.

5. Go into the living room and say to him, "Okay, I'm ready."

He will look you over and say, "You're going like *that*?" Your response should be, "Why not? I'm comfortable." Without missing a beat, he'll likely say "Great. Let's go." Warning: Before trying this, make sure you stash a scarf and some dark glasses in the car, in case you see anyone you know.

TRUTH OR CONSEQUENCES

I've noticed that probably the biggest difference between grandmothers and grandfathers is that, as a rule, grandmothers don't like fibbing to their grandkids unless it's for a good cause. Grand*fathers,* on the other hand, seem to think that it's part of their job to tell whoppers to their grandchildren whenever the opportunity presents itself. Fibbing and embellishing come naturally to men.

Imagine the following. . . .

SCENE 1

A granddaughter is in the kitchen, helping her grandmother bake cookies, when she notices something.

GRANDDAUGHTER: Grandma, what's that thing in your ear?

GRANDMOTHER: It's called a hearing aid, sweetie. And I wear it so I can hear you better. Sometimes when people get older, their ears don't work as well as when they were younger.

GRANDDAUGHTER: Oh.

SCENE 2

A granddaughter is on the sofa, coloring. She's sitting next to her grandfather, who closely watches a football game. She notices something.

GRANDDAUGHTER: Grandpa, what's that thing in your ear?

GRANDFATHER: That, beautiful little lady, is a secret transmitter so your grandpa can hear and talk to the football coach on the television and tell him what to do. (*Grandpa points to the coach on the sideline.*) See him there? The fat guy with the headphones on? He wears those so he can hear me. (*Grandfather yells at TV*) Throw it! (*The quarterback throws a pass. The granddaughter is amazed.*)

GRANDDAUGHTER: (*Awestruck*) Wow! He threw it just like you said! (*The grandfather nods proudly*) Is that why you yell at the TV?

GRANDFATHER: Exactly. But, ssshhhh; don't tell anyone, okay?

GRANDDAUGHTER: (*Whispers conspiratorially*) Okay.

I've been a witness to some of Mike's stories to the granddaughters, but following is one that came back to bite him.

When our granddaughter, Alexandra, was about five, she asked Mike if he had been in the army like her other grandpa.

"Nope. Air Force," Mike said proudly.

"Really?" Alex said, impressed. "Is flying scary?"

"Oh, yeah," said Mike.

I had to stifle a sarcastic laugh because I knew that the only thing he flew in the Air Force was an IBM Selectric in Springfield, Massachusetts.

"You have to be very brave to fly," Mike continued to the impressed five-year-old. "And handsome, too."

"*I'm* brave," she said. "I didn't cry last time when I got a shot. Could I go flying with you some time?" she asked.

"Yeah," I said. "Why don't you take Alex up into the ol' wild blue and show her how brave you are?"

"I'd like to, Alex," Mike said gravely. "But I'm not allowed to fly anymore."

"How come?"

"Yeah, how come?" I asked him, dying to see how he'd squirm out of this one.

"Well, you see . . ." Mike said, looking Alexandra squarely in the eyes. "Do you know what a covert operation is?"

She thought for a moment. "Isn't that when you have to go to a hospital?"

"Exactly," he said. "I had to stop flying when I went into the hospital."

"What was wrong with you?"

"Advanced Poughkeepsie-itis. I got it from flying way too brave." (FYI: We had just returned from Manhattan and upstate New York, and for some reason, "Poughkeepsie" had become a running joke with us.)

"Are you okay now?" Alex asked him with genuine concern.

"Yes I am, honey," Mike said. "Except sometimes I have to take naps. And when that happens, you should remind your grandmother here to be very nice to me, and let me sleep even if I snore and drool."

Alex nodded respectfully, kissed him, and ran off.

Within minutes, Mike had forgotten all about his tale. But apparently Alex hadn't, which we discovered when we attended one of her soccer games a year later.

Allow me a minute to tell you about our granddaughter, Alex. She is now six, and excels at every sport and physical activity she tries. She runs tirelessly from one end of the soccer field to the other, and is usually her team's leading scorer. Her mother recently enrolled her in a ballet class, and after the first session, her instructor was amazed that Alex had never danced before. Alex is a whirlwind of energy, and attacks everything she tries with vigor and joy.

I know I sound like a bragging grandma. And I am, because, you see, Alex was born with Cystic Fibrosis. It's a genetic disease that, so far, is without a cure. Hopefully, research will solve that soon, but until then, Alex is required to take breathing treatments and therapy twice a day to prevent mucous from forming in her lungs. But rather than pamper and coddle her, Alex's parents and sisters not only support her to the max, they also encourage her to participate in any activity she chooses.

It may sound odd to call Alexandra a lucky little girl, but that's the way we all see it. And I think she does, too.

Anyway, we were waiting for Alex's soccer game to begin when a swarthy, friendly guy about Mike's age walked up to us.

"Hey. You're Alexandra's grandfather, right?" he asked Mike.

"Sure am," Mike said.

"Bob Johnson," the man said. "Stephanie's grandpa," he explained, motioning to one of Alex's teammates.

"Nice to meet you, Bob," Mike said. "So what's up?"

"Just wanted to say 'hey' to a brother," Bob said, congenially. When he saw Mike's confused look, he continued. "89ᵗʰ Tac Wing, Pleiku, '67 and '68. Where were you?"

"Pardon?" Mike replied. I could tell that Mike feared Bob was likely a nut job.

"Alexandra told Stephanie that her grandpa used to fly, too," Bob said. "F–4s, right?"

Mike thought for a moment and then realized where this whole thing started. "Oh, no, sorry, Bob," Mike said, realizing that the "nut job" might just be none other than himself.

"You weren't in the Air Force?" Bob asked.

"Yeah, '66 to '70. But I worked in personnel," Mike confessed.

"Personnel? You were a desk jockey?" Bob asked dismissively.

"Yeah," Mike said. "I think what happened was . . ." He paused, trying to come up with some sort of plausible explanation. "You see, Bob," he started, "when I told Alex about my stint in the Air Force, she must've thought I said, 'I used to *fly*.' But actually, what I said was, 'I used to *file*.'"

Bob stared at Mike for a minute, then walked off as the game started.

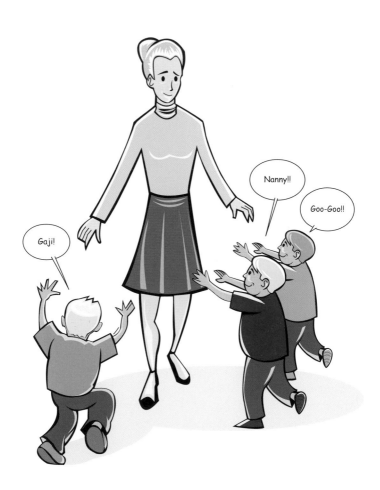

SEVEN

A GRANDMOTHER BY ANY OTHER NAME IS A "NANA," A "GRANDMA," OR EVEN A "GAJI"

Young Lars Kjernstrom lived in Minnesota. He was born into a large, loving, and multi-generational family whose men had long told a story of an amazing tradition accomplished by generations of rough-and-tumble male Kjernstroms.

As the story went, Lars' father, grandfather, and great-grandfather, all fishermen and hunters and barley farmers, were all able to walk on water on their 16th birthday. On that special day, they had each walked across the lake to the family cabin on the far side and been rewarded with their first alcoholic drink.

Lars, on the other hand, eschewed hunting and fishing and was more concerned about his grades and being the first in his family to go to college. He disliked even the smell of alcohol.

But when his 16th birthday came around, Lars felt it was his duty to uphold the tradition, so he asked his pal Sven to row him out to the middle of the lake. Lars stepped off . . . and almost drowned before Sven pulled him to safety.

Lars was embarrassed and confused, and was afraid to talk to his father, grandfather, or great-grandfather, fearing they'd mock him for being unable to carry on the family tradition.

So he went to his kindly grandmother, whom he loved very much and called "Bebo." "Bebo," he started, "it's my 16th birthday, and I tried to walk across the lake just like my father, his father, and his father before him. But I couldn't do it and fell in. What's wrong with me?"

Bebo Kjernstrom looked into his troubled eyes and knew she had to be honest with her grandson . . . he would have to handle the truth like a man. "You couldn't do it because your father, grandfather, and great-grandfather were born in January, when the lake is frozen, and you were born in July, you dumb ass."

Okay, so Lars' grandmother wasn't the most gentle of hearts, and neither was she born with the name "Bebo." In fact, she had gone the first forty-nine years of her life perfectly happy with being called by her given name, Beatrice Borgenson. But when Lars was about eleven months old, he stared up from his crib at his grandmother and said, "Goo-Goo!"

Lars' mother, Inga, was thrilled when she heard her baby son's pronouncement. "Goo-Goo," Inga said, excited. "Did you hear that, Beatrice? Lars just called you 'Goo-Goo!' To Inga, it was as if her brilliant child had just recited all the words to "Norwegian Wood."

Then Inga leaned into the crib and gently pinched her son's rosy cheeks. "You just gave your grandmother a new name, didn't you?"

And again Lars pointed at Beatrice and said, "Goo-Goo."

"See?" Inga crowed. "Well, it looks like you are officially 'Goo-Goo.'"

Beatrice stared at her daughter-in-law for a moment, and then said "Goo-Goo? No way, Jose."

Inga was stunned. "But that's what he wants to call you."

"I don't care if he wants to call me 'Sheena, Queen of the Jungle.' What kind of name is 'Goo-Goo'?"

"I think it's precious," Inga insisted.

"Yeah? Then let him call you 'Goo-Goo.'" Beatrice said. "Couldn't he just call me 'Grandma'?"

"No, my mom's already reserved that for herself," Inga informed her.

"Okay, how about 'Nana'?"

"Sorry, but that's what Jenny wants to be called." Jenny, who works the graveyard shift as fish-sniffer at a nearby cannery, is married to Beatrice's ex-husband, Randy, a professional downhill snowshoe racer.

Although Beatrice was just a little jealous that the other two grandmothers had already reserved their grandma names, she didn't really mind that "Grandma" and "Nana" were off the table. Beatrice had never really seen herself with a normal grandmother name.

Beatrice thought for a minute, and then blurted "Bebo!"

"Bebo?" Inga said. "What kind of name is that?"

"It's got a nice ring to it," Beatrice said, explaining that "Be" and Bo" combined the first two letters of her first and last name.

And so, for the next six weeks she trained her little grandson just like she had trained her parakeet when she was a little girl. Except, of course, for putting newspaper in his crib.

Then one day, after weeks of repetition, everything clicked; Lars looked into Beatrice's eyes and said, "Bebo."

And Bebo was thrilled.

Beatrice's husband, Murray, by comparison, got his new grandfather name the very same day that Beatrice had decided she wanted to be called, "Bebo." He was hold-ing the baby that evening when Lars looked at Murray and once again said, "Goo-Goo!"

"Goo-Goo!" Murray said exuberantly, unaware of what had happened earlier in the day. "Did you hear that, every-body? He called me 'Goo-Goo'! What a great name, eh?"

And for the past sixteen years, "Goo-Goo" has been proving, I suppose, the axiom that one woman's trash is another man's treasure.

My grandma name is "Gaji," and no, that isn't the same word used for an illegal crop popular in the Caribbean. "Gaji" came about when my first granddaughter had just started walking. For nearly two months, I had been after her to say "Grandma Jill." Each time I'd say it, she'd stare at me blankly, and every so often would show her displeasure at my haranguing by making her face all red and puffy and pooping in her diaper.

Then one day I was just about to give up and settle for something . . . anything . . . when she came out with "Gaaaa . . . jee . . ."

"What was that, honey?" I asked.

"Gaaaa . . . jee . . ." she repeated, this time pointing at me. I was puzzled at first, but then realized that with "Gaaaa," she was making the first sound of "grandma." (Okay, so she forgot the "R" but I had just changed her diaper and didn't want her to dirty it all over again because of my nitpick-ing.) And then came "jee," which was obviously a baby's way of making the "ji" sound. So there it was: "gaaa" for "grandma" and "jee" for "Jill."

Was this child brilliant or what? And that's why, for the past fourteen years, I have been known as "Gaji" to all four of our grandchildren . . . although the older ones now sometimes shorten it to "Gaj."

Mike, on the other hand, got his grandpa name when he was holding Sydni as a ten-month-old. She reached up, grabbed his ample, red, Irish nose and said, "Buh-Buh-Buh-Buh." But because that was too long to fit on his letterhead, Mike shortened it to "Buh-Buh," which he's been ever since. Although "Buh-Buh" lacks certain panache—it will likely serve him well should he ever be up for a writing job on a remake of "Gomer Pyle."

So here's a Grandma Rule for you: Although grandfathers seem perfectly content with whatever name they're given, grandmothers are often very particular about what they want to be called. However, if you're waiting for something like "Grandma Prettiest," or "Grandma Whose Rear End Doesn't Look At All Big In Those Jeans," it may take awhile.

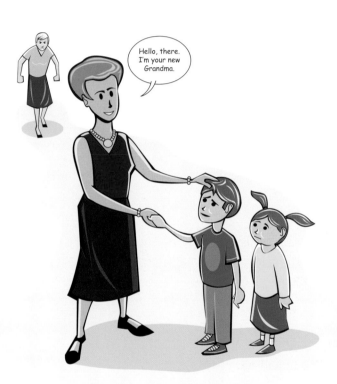

EIGHT

GRANDMA OR NOT?

"Grandmother" isn't just a title, it's also a state of mind cherished by millions of women known as "Grandma," or "Nana," or "Gaji," or whatever name they've been given.

Others cherish it not quite as much.

Take my friend, Jane. She just celebrated her 53rd birthday, and everyone agrees that she doesn't look a day over forty. Without the help of surgery, dieting, or Suzanne Somers, Jane has an absolutely stunning body, and has been a size 6 since she was fifteen. Some of my jealous friends say this is because Jane never bore children, but I suspect Jane could've had more kids than the Osmonds and still look terrific. Her straight teeth are sparkling white, her light olive skin is smoother than a Lionel Richie ballad, and her breasts are still exactly where God put them. She is also extremely intelligent and successful.

Jane is, quite simply, the kind of woman I love to hate. If only she weren't so darn nice.

But perfection took a blow several years ago when Jane was blindsided by her husband, who suddenly left her. In a cruel and ironic twist of fate, it was for an older woman.

Jane spent over a week locked in her house and cutting herself off from all her friends. We called her daily, but she didn't answer or return any of our phone calls. Even trips to her house went unanswered. Then one day my phone rang and it was Jane, asking me to come over. She said she called *me* because I'd gone through a divorce myself, because I was a good listener, and because I made killer margaritas.

I rang the bell and when Jane answered, I saw standing in front of me a woman who'd been unceremoniously dumped, who'd spent the last ten days locked in her house, eating nothing but Haagen-Dazs, wearing no makeup, not even showering.

A woman who looked . . . absolutely terrific. Damn!

Jane fell into my arms and began bawling. But a quart of Cuervo later, she was feeling a little better.

"Oh well," she reasoned blearily, "if my marriage has to be on the rocks, I'm glad the margaritas are, too."

As the months rolled by, Jane gradually began recapturing her joy, and eventually began dating—something she hadn't done in over fifteen years. It was awkward at first, but after a string of losers—including one guy who insisted she call him "Colonel," even though he had never been in the military—Jane met a really terrific guy her age. She and Neil have been together for six years, married for two.

After a few dates, Jane met Neil's four-year-old grandson, Teddy, at a family barbecue. Jane thought that Teddy was cute, even though he always seemed to have dirty hands and a runny nose, a combo that didn't sit well with her white linen slacks. But Jane liked the little rascal, and thought it was cute how Teddy called her and Neil "Jane and Pop-Pop."

Jane and Neil were married two years later in a small wedding in Neil's backyard. As soon as the ceremony concluded, and they were enjoying their first marital kiss, Teddy—by then a rambunctious six-year-old, ran up to Jane and cried, "Grandma!"

Jane was stunned. "Grandma?" What was he talking about? Then Teddy threw his deviled-egg covered hands around her and her white satin dress, and repeated himself. "You're my grandma now!" he squealed.

Uh-oh, she thought.

Jane didn't want to make an issue of it then. But later, while everyone was dancing the Funky Chicken, she pulled Teddy aside for a little chat. Jane never told me exactly what they talked about, but later said it was very loving and honest conversation and that both she and little Teddy learned something that night.

He would never again call her "Grandma."

And she would never again wear white when he was around.

As a contrast to Jane's story, let's take a look at Mike's friend, "Calvin," a fifty-eight-year-old divorced CPA with grown children. Calvin also has two lovely grandchildren, whom he loves dearly.

Following his divorce, Calvin's self-esteem went into a downward spiral, and even though he doesn't drink alcohol, he began frequenting bars. Calvin's rationale for this unusual behavior was this: If he had to feel miserable, it was more satisfying to share it with others. One night, as he was pounding back his fifth ginger ale, he caught the eye of Greta, a fifty-eight-year-old Austrian-born divorcee and herself a grandmother. She moved to the stool next to him and began chatting him up, and after listening to his morose story and hearing him constantly refer to himself as a hapless loser, Greta had to agree with his assessment.

But as a restorer of used furniture, Greta loved reclamation projects. So after a few more "chance" encounters at this bar, Greta invited Calvin for dinner. This led to another dinner, and then another as Greta gradually began rehabilitating Calvin's self-worth—first with words of flattery, then by hand-holding, and finally by showing him her recent boob job, compliments of an alimony settlement from her fourth husband.

Needless to say, Calvin was smitten, and threw his accountant's caution to the wind by eloping with Greta to Las Vegas, where their wedding was performed by a male Streisand impersonator and witnessed by two acrobats from Cirque du Soleil.

After a whirlwind honeymoon, they returned home and Calvin was soon introduced to Greta's three-year-old grandson, Dirk.

"Hello, Dirk, sweetie. I want you to meet your new Grandpa Calvin," Greta said.

This caught Calvin off guard, as he certainly didn't think of himself as this child's grandfather. And apparently neither did Dirk, who studied Calvin and then called him "Doo-doo head."

Next, Dirk hurled a large Lincoln Log at Calvin's balding noggin.

"Isn't he cute?" Greta asked Calvin.

"Oh, yes," said Calvin, not wanting to upset his new bride. "Now, do you suppose you could get me a Band-Aid?"

Calvin later explained to Greta that he wasn't really Dirk's grandfather, adding that he already had two grandchildren of his own and was quite satisfied with that.

"Of course you're Dirk's grandpa," insisted Greta. "Just like I'm your grandchildren's new grandma."

Greta's bold and uninvited proprietorship of *his* grandchildren irked Calvin a bit, and he could only imagine how his family would react if Greta were to saunter up to his grandkids and say, "Come give your new granny a big kiss!" Calvin thought about his granddaughter's upcoming first grade talent show. A family party was planned afterward, and he had been privately anguishing over whether to bring Greta to meet his children, his grandchildren . . . and Barb, his ex-wife.

Calvin reflected on how having grandchildren had managed to narrow the divide between him and Barb, feeling that their relationship had progressed from unabated dislike to one of frigid civility.

Just like the last few years of their marriage.

Calvin wondered if he, in good conscience, should take Greta to the gathering knowing that Barb, who was absolutely gaga over her only grandkids, would likely go ballistic if Greta tried to claim even the slightest bit of ownership of them. Barb was a professional landscape architect, which meant she had easy access to any number of sharp tools. It could get ugly.

Calvin decided Greta should go.

At the family party, Greta did, in fact, ignore Calvin's warnings and introduced herself as Calvin's grandkids' new grandma.

But only once because Barb immediately yanked her aside and explained that if she ever heard that come out of Greta's cap-toothed mouth again, she would stuff it with a handful of mulching material.

It wasn't long after that that Calvin realized the mistake of his impulsive marriage. And now, two years later, Greta is just a footnote to Calvin's life and is remembered as "the witch who was briefly married to Grandpa."

Praise the Lord and pass the ginger ale.

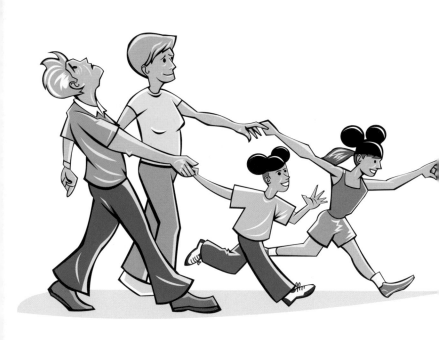

NINE

GRANDMAS HERE, GRANDMAS THERE, GRANDMAS, GRANDMAS, EVERYWHERE

Most grandmothers fall into one of two categories: 1) those who live near their grandchildren, and 2) those who don't. If you and your grandchildren are separated by great distances, you know that "absence makes the heart grow fonder." If you live close to your grandkids, you've learned that "nearness makes the house grow messier."

These two groups are much like airport parking lots: long term and short term. A grandmother who lives nearby her grandkids is the short term lot—she's used much more often, but the stays are usually relatively brief. The long-term grandma doesn't see her grandchildren nearly as often. But when she does, their stays usually last for days, sometimes (gulp!) weeks. The long-term grandma is normally used by parents who want to park their kids while they go on vacation. And although the job requirements—to love, nurture, and care for our grandchildren—is the same for both groups, the responsibilities and demands are quite different.

SHORT-TERM GRANDMOTHERS

If you live near your grandchildren, think of yourself as a fireman . . . you are available whenever duty calls. And even when you think you're officially off duty, experience has taught you that a four-alarm emergency could arise at any moment, and you'll be called into action without much warning. (These "emergencies" include a baby-sitter canceling at the last moment, parents coming down with the flu, or scoring last minute tickets to a Barenaked Ladies concert.) And like a fireman, you know that the only way to *really* be off duty is to take a vacation to a land far, far away, where the cries of "Hey, Grandma, look at this!" or "Nana, he hit me!" are replaced by the sound of gently swaying palm fronds. Instead of grandchildren screaming, "I want my toy!" you will be saying, "I want my mai-tai!"

Because we are a six-hour drive from our grandchildren, I'm sometimes envious of my grandmother pals who get to see their grandkids almost every day. But notice that I said "sometimes," which does not mean "always."

Consider our friends Bart and Sherry, whom we've known for years, way before any of us became grandparents. Our lives pretty much traveled the same path: we had children, raised children, educated children, said good-bye to children, changed the locks before children knew what hit them. And like us, it didn't take Bart and Sherry long to get used to the lovely concepts of lower food bills, full gas tanks, and 24/7 bathroom availability. They redecorated their entire home, converting one of their kids' rooms into an office for Bart, and the other into an art studio for Sherry, even though Bart had a corner office at work, and the only art Sherry had done in years was playing Pictionary.

They had a huge garage sale and got rid of all the clutter they'd accumulated over twenty-three years of parenting, and from then on, their house was always spotless, never so much as a cushion out of place. Best of all, Sherry and

I started tennis lessons, trying to reacquaint ourselves with the sport we'd both enjoyed in our younger days.

When Chloe, their first granddaughter, was born, Bart and Sherry were understandably over-the-moon; and since their son, Steve, and daughter-in-law, Tina, lived only a few miles away, they'd be able to see their beautiful little girl whenever they wanted. Tina's parents came out from Vermont to pitch in for the first two weeks, and then Sherry took over. As I watched her feed her newborn granddaughter one day, give her a bath the next, and wipe vomited formula from her blouse the day after that, I wished my grandkids lived closer.

Then, after nine weeks of maternity leave, it was time for Tina to return to her bank V.P. position. This is a stressful time for all new parents, but Steve and Tina were soothed because they'd found a wonderful, nurturing environment for child care. In a proclamation usually reserved for one being awarded a Nobel Prize, or at least winning the lottery, they announced that their two-month-old daughter had been accepted into the New Age preschool called The Akidemy. Furthermore, they boasted that Chloe gained admission based on her successful "intake interview" with the school's headmaster.

Even Chloe's grandparents rolled their eyes at this one. "Intake interview? For a two-month-old?" Bart said, shaking his head.

Although The Akidemy was a unique place, there was one drawback. Because of her age, Chloe would only be able to attend three days a week. "To be accepted as a full-time student," their brochure read, "a child must be eighteen months old. . . . " Talk about age discrimination. But what this meant was that Steve and Tina needed to find someone to care for Chloe for the two remaining weekdays.

They researched and interviewed extensively, but by the time Tina had to return to work, they'd still not found anyone they considered suitable to care for their infant daughter.

So, of course, Sherry volunteered. "It's just two days a week," she told me with a brave smile. "And only until they find someone they like."

The initial changes in Sherry's spotless house were small and gradual: a pink baby blanket carelessly tossed over the back of her brand new sofa . . . the unmistakable aroma of pureed carrots wafting from the microwave . . . a baby's car seat always parked near the front door . . . a plastic bath tub on the kitchen counter.

And it wasn't long before a crib was planted squarely in the middle of Sherry's art studio. Then, a playpen and a huge *Finding Nemo* toy box appeared in Bart's home office. Sherry had to stop her tennis lessons; the only serving she was doing involved a jar of Gerber's. And the four of us have had to limit our frequent dinners out together to weekends only; Sherry was simply too exhausted during the week.

But she continues on cheerfully, and her granddaughter simply adores her. And although Sherry keeps nudging the kids to find someone to replace her, she knows that even if they don't, it's only nine more months before Chloe will be going to The Akidemy full time.

But overall, Sherry having all this time with her granddaughter has been a good thing for everyone—including me. You see, I've continued my tennis lessons. And when Sherry returns . . . I am gonna make her weep!

LONG-TERM GRANDMOTHERS

Because short-term grandmothers like Sherry get to see their grandkids whenever they like, they don't feel the need to make every visit special or memorable. But for us long-termers, it's a big deal when we see our grandkids, especially when they come to visit us.

Several years ago, our two oldest granddaughters, Sydni and Samantha, came to Southern California to stay with us while their parents went on a short cruise to the Mexican Riviera to celebrate their tenth wedding anniversary. The girls, who were nine and five at the time, would be with us for four full days—the longest they'd ever stayed anywhere without their parents—and we were excited about having all that time with them. Ron and Dionn would drop them with us Thursday morning, then head off to their cruise ship and return on Sunday.

Wednesday afternoon, I went to the supermarket and bought a variety of cereals, two dozen frozen waffles, syrup, snacks, bologna, milk, ice cream, soda, and whatever else their mother said they shouldn't have.

Wednesday night, Mike and I made out a list of all the fun things we were going to cram into the short time our grandchildren were with us. That's what long-term grandparents do.

The following is our recorded log of that four day visit. . . .

Thursday 12:30 P.M. Grandkids arrive with their parents, who immediately hand us their "Don't" list, which is a directory of forbidden pleasures that their children should not enjoy while staying with us. Included on the list are no junk food, no staying up past nine, no swimming within thirty minutes after meals, and no watching television while they're eating.

Thursday 12:45 P.M. After kissing their beautiful daughters good-bye, their parents drive off down the street. The girls and Mike wave good-bye. I tear up the "Don't" list.

Thursday 1:15 P.M. Sydni and Samantha eat their lunch of corn dogs, Fritos, and Oreos while watching *Hannah Montana*.

Thursday 1:18 P.M. Girls and I jump into the pool. We swim for three hours. Neither child suffers cramps or ingests huge amounts of chlorinated water. I get pinkeye.

Thursday 5:41 P.M. We go to an early movie to see "Winged Migration," an Oscar-nominated, French documentary about birds flying to the Arctic. The girls seem to enjoy it, but when we visit them six months later and offer to take them to another movie, Samantha says, "Okay, but it's not another one about French ducks, is it?"

Thursday 7:15 P.M. After the movie, the girls are full of popcorn and Red Vines, so instead of dinner, we go to Baskin-Robbins. We know that dairy products are an important part of young children's diets.

Thursday 8:42 P.M. Girls are changed into their pajamas and ready for their 9:00 bedtime. I suggest we play cards for awhile.

Thursday 10:36 P.M. After twelve games of Old Maid and ten of Crazy Eights, we decide to call it a night.

Thursday 10:50 P.M. The girls are asleep and Mike and I are scheduling tomorrow's activities when the phone rings. It's Ron and Dionn calling from the ship. They stop singing "Tequila Sunrise" long enough to ask if they woke us. "Of course you woke us," I lied. "We went to bed at 9:00 with the girls." Hearing this, they blubbered, "We love you guys sooooo much!" They seemed to be having a good time; I suspected they wouldn't be waking up as early in the morning as we would.

Friday 8:00 A.M. I'm helping the girls get showered; Mike's in the kitchen making his "secret recipe" blueberry-chocolate-chip pancakes, a special treat he made for his kids forty-five years earlier. He's doing it from memory. "No better way to start the day than with homemade pancakes!" he says.

Friday 8:30 A.M. We make an unplanned stop at Denny's for breakfast.

Friday 10:30 A.M. We arrive at Disneyland early, wanting to be the first ones in. Apparently we're not the only ones with that plan, as we have to park so far away that we may actually be closer to Disney World.

Friday 11:00 A.M. Gates open and I have words with an extremely aggressive lady who nearly flattens our granddaughters in her haste to get to the nearest food court.

Friday 11:15 A.M. to 5:10 P.M. The ride lines are long, but we manage to go on It's a Small World three times, The Matterhorn twice, Space Mountain, Tarzan's Treehouse, and Splash Mountain. The girls take pictures with Mickey, Minnie, Goofy, and Snow White. Mike takes two puffs from his inhaler.

Friday 5:30 P.M. Even though we had a healthy lunch of nachos and chicken fingers, the girls are hungry again and we take a welcome break for dinner, where we have hamburgers, fries, sodas, and ice cream. When the bill arrives and Mike sees the total, he has to use his inhaler again.

Friday 6:27 P.M. As we head out for the *Finding Nemo* Submarine Adventure and The Jungle Cruise, it seems that dinner has reenergized Sydni and Samantha, who now want to run everywhere full speed. I try to keep up with them, but when my cell phone rings, I appoint Mike as their wrangler. I answer, and it's my son-in-law calling from a cantina in Cabo San Lucas, their ship's first stop.

"How's Disneyland?" he asked giddily.

"Great," I told him. "The girls are being perfect angels," I said, looking off to see Mike scolding Syd for wiping her nose on Sam's new Tinkerbell T-shirt.

"Good, Jill," he said. "Could you hold on for a minute?" Then he covered the phone and called off to someone,

"Yo, Paco! Una mas sangria, por favor!" Then we got disconnected.

Friday 10:36 P.M. After going on virtually every ride in the park and staying for Festival of Lights *and* the fireworks, we drag ourselves down Main Street toward the exit. But first, we stop to buy Mickey Mouse hats, Cinderella magic wands, stuffed Jiminy Crickets, and other souvenirs to guarantee that our granddaughters will always remember this magical day with their Gaji and Buh-Buh.

Friday 10:49 P.M. As we leave Disneyland, two performers dressed as Doc and Bashful say to us, "Thank you for coming to the happiest place on earth!" Mike whispers to me that if he sees one more jovial little dwarf tonight, he's gonna smack him all the way into tomorrow.

Saturday 12:37 A.M. We arrive home with the girls sound asleep in the back seat. Mike pulls a muscle in his back lifting Syd. I carry Sam and we deposit them in their beds, fully dressed. Mike hobbles into the bathroom for a double dose of Advil, and I tuck the girls in for the night. Then as I creep out, Sydni pries her eyes open. "I love you, Gaj," she says. "Me, too," mumbles Samantha, too exhausted to open her eyes. All of a sudden, I don't feel tired anymore.

Saturday 8:14 A.M. We are all still asleep when the phone rings. It's a representative from the Credit Card Fraud Division of American Express to inquire about a significant amount of activity over the past 24 hours that didn't match our normal spending patterns.

"Disneyland?" Mike asked.

"That's right."

"No, all of that was us," he said.

"Wow!" the representative said, impressed. "So your card hasn't been stolen?"

"I wish," he said. Then he thanked her for her vigilance and said good-bye. He hung the phone up quietly, not wanting to wake up the girls so we could grab a bit more rest before checking to see if our legs still worked.

Saturday 8:16 A.M. No such luck. They both come into our bedroom wearing their bathing suits. "We're ready to go!"

"Go where?" I asked.

"The beach, remember? You said we were going to take a picnic and then rent bikes. Can I rent a red one?"

"I want blue!" said her sister.

NOTE: IMPORTANT GRANDMA RULE: If you live near your grandchildren and see them often, you can barter your way out of situations like these by offering an alternative. "I know we said we'd go to the beach today, but let's do it tomorrow . . . or the day after. Today, let's make cookies!"

But if you are a long-term grandma, there's often no "tomorrow" or "the next day." And worse, your grandchildren know this, and they will resort any tactic—alligator tears and quivering lower lips included—to their advantage. Therefore, you have absolutely no wiggle room in situations like these, unless you are a grandparent who is extremely intelligent and creative. Or rich.

Saturday 11:37 A.M. We pull into the beach parking lot and begin unloading the car. Mike wonders if we could steal someone's handicapped placard.

Saturday 2:30 P.M. The girls have been frolicking in the surf since we arrived. It's a hot and sunny day and we're careful to slather them with SPF 30. Mike insists on using SPF 4 because, "I'm a 'sun' guy; I grew up at the beach, remember?"

Saturday 3:15 P.M. to 7:30 P.M. We rent four bicycles to ride from one end of the beach bike path to the other and back again. Mike brings up the rear and twice volunteers to stop, saying he doesn't want to slow us down, and suggesting that we continue on and he'd meet us on our way back. Each of these offers, coincidentally, comes when he spots a beach bar and grill featuring thonged waitresses. But his granddaughters guilt him into making the full round-trip, a distance we later learn was fourteen miles.

Saturday 7:42 P.M. The bikes are returned and the car is loaded. The four of us sit on the beach, cuddling in a large blanket as we watch the sun set over the water. In the fading light, I notice that Mike's face is the color of a glowing charcoal briquette.

Saturday 9:15 P.M. Back home now, the girls and I are dressed for bed, watching a rerun of "That's So Raven." Apparently they've seen this episode countless times, and recite every line of dialogue. I, on the other hand, have barely enough energy to open my lips to sip my oxygenated energy drink. Mike is in the bathtub, soaking in a mixture of cold water and vinegar. Apparently SPF 4 is fine when you're fifteen. But when you're fifty-one? Not so much . . .

Sunday 8:47 A.M. The girls come into our room and crawl in bed with us. Sam asks Mike why he smells like salad dressing.

Sunday 11:29 A.M. Mike and I sit under an umbrella and watch our granddaughters swimming and diving in our pool. They beg us to join them, but after two-plus days of non-stop activities, we are both absolutely exhausted. The only dive we want to take is into our bed. I check my watch. Still four more hours until their parents return.

Sunday 2:30 P.M. I'm shopping with the girls. I figure since we boosted the economy of Disneyland, why not do the same for the mall?

Sunday 2:32 p.m. Mike is on the sofa, nodding off in front of a football game, when a news flash gets his attention. A cruise ship on its way back to Los Angeles from Mexico was struck by a small fishing boat. There are no injuries, but the liner will be diverted to San Diego for a safety check and won't return to Los Angeles until Monday morning.

Sunday 2:47 p.m. After several frantic calls to every cruise line that sails from L.A. to Mexico, Mike learns that the kids' boat was not the one involved in the accident and that they'll be back as scheduled. He celebrates by moistening his sunburned chest with yet another coat of aloe.

Sunday 4:57 p.m. We stand in our driveway waving good-bye to our two beautiful granddaughters as they head off on their long drive home with their parents. As their car disappears around the corner, I take Mike's hand and we hobble back toward our house, wearing sombreros with our names stitched on them.

Sunday 7:30 p.m. After a dinner of soup and scotch, we decide it's way past our bedtime. On the way to our room, Mike remembers that he has a breakfast meeting in the morning with his agent—a grandfather whose grandkids live right around the corner from him.

Sunday 7:35 p.m. "Hi, Lew," Mike says into the phone. "Listen, I need to reschedule our breakfast in the morning. See, we had the grandkids this weekend and . . . What? Wore me out? No way! The truth is . . . Did you see that thing on the news about the cruise ship and the fishing boat? Well, their parents were on that ship and won't be back until tomorrow, so we get to keep 'em another day! I'm taking them roller skating in the morning! Yeah, you're right. We *are* lucky!"

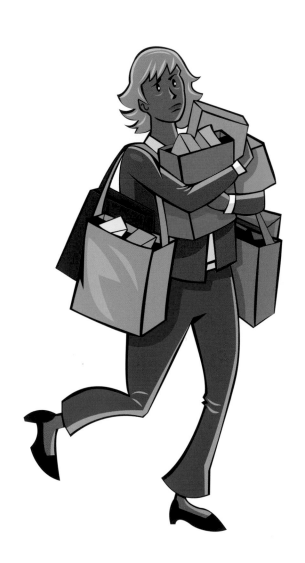

TEN

TALKIN' 'BOUT MY GENERATION

As an active participant in three generations of mothering in my family—as a daughter, mother, and grandmother—here's what I've learned about each:

As a daughter, you *think* you know everything.

As a mother, you *know* you know everything.

As a grandmother, you know they really don't know diddley.

You also know that if Necessity is the Mother of Invention, then Experience is the Grandmother.

And this experience has taught you not to offer unsolicited advice on child care unless you're asked. And although it will probably be awhile before you *are* asked, give it time, because it will happen. Meanwhile, just try to smile when your children think they've got all the parenting answers. Remember that your grandchild's extremely wise mother is your daughter, who not all that long ago tried to hard boil an egg in the microwave. Or the father is your son, who, only a few years back, thought it was oh-so-cool to walk through the mall with his shorts belted around his knees.

Experience has also taught you that no matter how many parenting guides your children read, or how much time they spend online at howtobethebestparentsever.com, they will eventually come to realize that, while a little

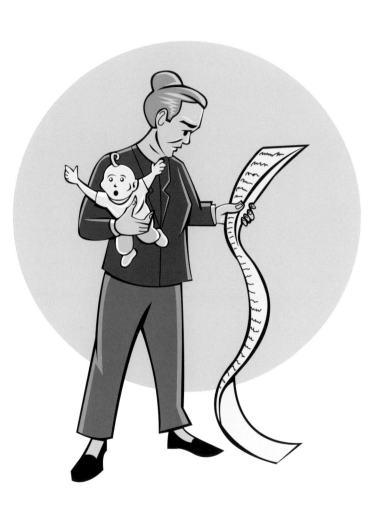

knowledge is a fine thing, 95 percent of good parenting is based on instinct and common sense.

And that the other 5 percent is pure luck.

And while the value of experience is obvious to any grandmother, it's not always evident to our children, who are often under the impression that they are the first people ever to raise a child. This may explain why many of them think it's necessary—when a grandma babysits for the first time—to leave her with a set of instructions more detailed than a bomb defusing manual.

When I was a young mom, I often called on my mother to babysit, reasoning that if she could survive the difficult task of raising me without either of us sustaining serious injury, a few hours of watching my eleven month-old daughter would be a snap.

"Hi, Mom, thanks for coming. Dee's sleeping," I said when she showed up, right on time.

"Okay," she answered, sitting down and switching on *The Mike Douglas Show.*

"There are two fresh bottles in the fridge, and her food's on the counter," I told her.

"Gotcha," she said as Mike Douglas introduced his next guest.

"She'll probably wake up soon."

"I'll hear her," Mom said confidently, in an era when baby monitors had a different name: ears.

"Oh, look! Fred Astaire!" she said. "They don't make dancers like that anymore."

"Okay," I said, opening the door to leave. "See you in a few hours."

Mom answered with a wave, not wanting to miss a word of her show. And I left with the confidence that whatever came up while I was gone, mom would know exactly what to do. That's because I trusted her experience.

And sure enough, when I got home, my mother had Dee on her lap. They were playing pat-a-cake, and Dee was howling with delight. She had on a nice clean outfit, and mom had obviously given her a bath.

"You didn't have to do all that," I told her.

"Oh, we had fun," she said. "She had just a touch of diaper rash, so I put some cream on it."

Imagine . . . all that without instructions.

I thought back to those times recently when Mischon and Kevin asked if I could travel to Northern California and pitch in with some temporary child care for our beautiful eleven-month-old granddaughter, Claire. Of course, I was thrilled at the opportunity to spend three full days with my newest granddaughter while her parents were at work. I should also tell you that Mischon and Kevin are wonderful and attentive young parents; Claire is very lucky to have them.

I arrived late Sunday and Claire was already in bed for the night. Mischon informed me that they leave for work around 6 A.M. to beat the traffic into San Francisco, so I should plan to be up around 5:30. After giving me a rundown on stroller operation and showing me all of Claire's food, we called it a day.

When my alarm went off the next morning, I sprung upright in bed thinking "Where am I?" and "Why am I there at 5:15?" Once I got my bearings, I dressed and brushed my teeth; that's when I heard Claire cooing in her crib.

Kevin had already left for work, and Mischon was getting dressed, so I took Claire from her crib and hugged her, kissed her, and hugged her some more, until I sensed it was time for a new diaper. I sang to her while I changed her, and she stared up at me with a big smile. Then I lifted her from the changing table . . . and hugged her even more.

"She may need a new diaper," Mischon said from the bedroom doorway, towel drying her hair.

"I already changed her," I said.

"All right, Mom! Way to go!" Mischon had such incredible amazement in her voice, it was as if I'd just solved a Rubik's Cube on my first try. Blindfolded.

Then I put a nice new outfit on Claire for her first full day with her Gaji. When we got to the kitchen, Mischon was ready to go.

"I've got her bottle in the warmer," she said.

"The what?"

"The bottle warmer," Mischon explained, pointing to an appliance on the counter. "Didn't you have one of those?"

When I explained that my bottle warmer was a pot of boiling water on the stove, I could see that her confidence in my ability to care for a child dropped a notch or so.

"It's set at 97 degrees," she explained. "They say that's a good temperature. It'll beep when it's ready."

"Oh, right," I said, wondering who "they" were.

"Okay, well, I guess I better get going," Mischon said as she gave Claire a huge kiss. "Be good for Gaji," she added.

Then as she headed for the door, she remembered one more thing. "Kevin jotted down a few notes to help you out," she said, pointing to a sheet of paper on the table. Then, when she said "See you later," I noticed a bit of concern in her voice.

"Don't worry, we'll be fine," I reassured her.

Mischon forced a smile, then looked at Claire as though this could very well be the last time she'd ever see her daughter in such good working condition. Then she left, and Claire and I were all alone. As I waited for the bottle warmer to beep at the "perfect" temperature, I decided to go over Kevin's page of notes. The paper was crammed with very neat—but small—printing, and I wondered how many instructions there could be for one nine-hour shift of babysitting. So imagine my surprise when I picked up the paper to find two more sheets stapled to it—three pages—all in the same small printing.

Kevin's instructions covered—down to the precise minute—everything except how many breaths Claire should take per minute, and what we should do if attacked by Canada. There were directives on nap times, feeding schedules, diaper changing, and baby's wardrobe from the time we woke up until Claire's parents returned home at 5 P.M. Here are just some of the list's highlights:

"Breakfast. Use high chair and bib." (*Gee, ya think?*)

"After buckling her in, attach tray." (*Wow! So that's how those things work!*)

"If she shows no interest in finger food, you can feed her by hand." (*Hey, there's a concept.*)

"After a bottle, I will stand up with her. She puts her head on my shoulder and we sway gently. After 1-2 minutes, I put her in the crib." (*No sardonic comment on this one. I just wanted to brag about what a sweet guy and tender dad my son-in-law is.*)

"Lunch. Use same high chair routine as breakfast." (*Okay, but at my age I hope I can remember what that was*).

"If she begins dropping her food on the floor, this is either a sign that she's almost finished, or just playing." (*Or perhaps she's trying to tell* you, "*It's tofu. What would* you *do with it?*")

But here's my favorite:

"Be careful when you put her on the diaper table so she doesn't fall off." (*You mean I have watch for stuff like that? Jeez, how much are you paying me?*)

In spite of my presumed complete ineptitude, Claire and I had three wonderful days together . . . And when her parents left for work on the third morning, any hesitation they'd had on day one was gone.

I must admit that Kevin's notes were amazingly helpful and insightful, and I followed them to the letter each day.

But I did add one thing of my own. Every afternoon, right before Kevin and Mischon got home from work, I'd give Claire a bath and dress her in a fresh new outfit. Then she and I would sit in the rocking chair together. And when her parents walked in, there we were . . . playing pat-a-cake, with Claire laughing that beautiful baby laugh.

And for that . . . Thanks, Mom.

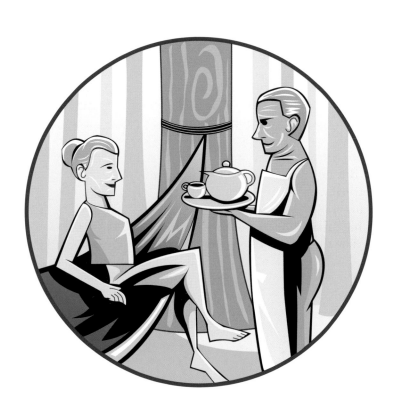

ELEVEN

COFFEE, TEA, OR GRANNY?

When we recall our grandmothers, I suspect many of us have similar associations . . . furniture with protective plastic, odors of suspicious origin, and dishes containing hard candy that hadn't been touched since the Coolidge administration.

But never did I associate my grandmother with sexual intimacy. Imagining Buzzie sleeping with her seventy-four-year-old handyman would be as disquieting as imagining Julia Roberts sleeping with Ernest Borgnine.

The truth is, of course, that our grandmothers were likely quite sensual in their day. But by the time we got to know them, they were too old for our child's eyes to see them in that context. And proper grandmothers never discuss their past or current sexual experiences.

Grandfathers seem to have the patent on that.

So I asked several of my friends if they had ever thought of their grandmothers and grandfathers having sex. Most of them shuddered and thought the entire notion was "creepy."

But not all of them.

Our good friend Denise is a warm-hearted and march-to-her-own-drummer businesswoman whose memories of her "Grandma and Grandpa B" include hand-holding, frequent kissing, and playful patting.

Like many of us who were trying to rush into puberty a few years before our bodies got there, Denise was eleven years old when she decided she needed the services of a brassiere, even though she was as flat as the prairie surrounding her small Texas town. When Denise mentioned this to her grandparents, they agreed wholeheartedly and soon Denise and Grandma B were on their way to the local department store to buy Denise her first bra . . . at least three years ahead of time.

Apparently not just any bra would do, and when Denise spotted a bright red, lace number, she just had to have it. Once again, Grandma B agreed, saying it was a perfect choice for such a beautiful little girl. Thrilled, Denise ran into the changing room and put on the fire engine-colored bra under the white cotton uniform blouse of Our Lady of Peace grammar school.

Needless to say, the next day Denise was the talk of the playground. She was so pleased with her bra that she wore it to school every day.

She even wore it on weekends and when she marched in her town's annual Fourth of July Parade.

"For the parade, Grandma B got me an outfit of blue satin shorts, a white tank top that said MISS AMERICA, and a pair of candy-apple red, high-heeled pumps," Denise told me. "With my red bra underneath, I twirled my baton down Main Street, proud as could be."

But halfway through the three-block parade route, Denise broke a heel on one of her red shoes and was unable to continue. She was heartbroken.

"What happened, honey?" Grandma B said, running into the street.

"My shoe broke," Denise sobbed. "I can't be in the parade anymore."

"Nonsense," said Grandma B; and then she quickly took Denise back to the store to buy another pair of red pumps.

But by the time they got back, the event had ended. Denise was crestfallen.

"Shoot," she said to her grandmother. "The parade's over."

"Over?" Grandma B asked, surprised. "The parade's never over. Because you see, sweetie, you are the parade."

Then Grandma B arranged for the local traffic cop to stop cars momentarily so Denise could complete the route.

And Denise did. And as she marched down the remaining one-and-a-half blocks of Main Street all by herself, twirling her baton, she felt way more important than any Miss America.

Then there's my friend Grace, who told me a story about her grandmother, Bobbi, who lived until age ninety-two, when Grace was well into her thirties. In her youth, Bobbi had been a professional dancer, appearing in films alongside such stars as Mickey Rooney, Judy Garland, and Delores del Rio. And it was around this time that Bobbi met a dashing young magician named Hobart the Wondrous. They fell madly in love and were soon joined in a marriage that lasted fifty-seven passionate years, until Hobart passed away in 1980.

Grace was very close to her grandparents, and on the day she received her acceptance letter to college, decided to drive over to their house and surprise them with the good news. Their isolated home was set in a grove of thick oaks, and as Grace walked toward their front door, she heard opera music blaring from the backyard deck. She went around to the rear of the house to investigate, but stopped short when she saw what was going on. Her seventy-two-year-old grandmother was lying on a hammock, wearing a sheer negligee that had been seductively lowered to her waist, while Hobart served her tea from a silver tray. And what's more . . . Hobart the Wondrous was wearing nothing more than one of Bobbi's full aprons, untied in the rear.

Grace turned away, but heard her grandfather say to her grandmother, "Tea, madame?"

"Tea? Oh, I'd rather have some of thee!" Bobbi said to Hobart. Grace couldn't help another peek, and saw Bobbi setting the tray aside and pulling her seventy-five-year-old husband onto the hammock atop her.

Grace was understandably flummoxed, and hurried back to her car. She closed her door and before she could start her motor, her initial shock gave way to uncontrollable laughter. *Imagine that*! she thought. Then she heard herself saying, "Way to go, Grandma and Grandpa. Rock on!"

Grace drove around for awhile to give them time to . . . whatever . . . and then stopped to call her grandparents from a nearby pay phone. Hobart answered.

"Hi, Grandpa. I'm not far from you guys and I thought maybe I'd stop by."

"Excellent, please do," said her grandfather. "We were just enjoying a little cup of tea!"

I know that my reaction to hearing this story as a grandma is completely different than what it would have been had I heard it as a child. Although our grandchildren will probably never consider such a "creepy" thought, of course their grandparents enjoy "a little cup of tea" every so often.

And it's not just my married grandmother friends who enjoy a little swing in the hammock now and then. A number of them are still dating—or trying to—like my free-spirited friend, Donna, who is truly one-of-a-kind. A while back, she called to tell me that she'd just joined an online dating service, and asked if I'd come over after dinner and help her weed through the male candidates to find her a date for an upcoming wedding.

"Sure, I'd love to," I told her. Then I expressed my surprise that Donna, an attractive and sexy grandmother of two, would have any trouble at all meeting men.

"You have no idea what it's like out there," she said over the phone. "I've tried networking, dance classes . . . Hell, I even joined a damn church. You don't know how lucky you are to have such a great husband."

As if on cue, Mike trudged in from the backyard, where he'd been trying to repair a broken sprinkler head. He was carrying his entire tool collection, which is limited to a large screwdriver and a pair of pliers. He was wearing ripped shorts, his old sneakers were caked in mud, and his dark T-shirt was covered in what appeared to be whipped cream.

"Can't fix it," he said. Then, as he left muddy footprints across the kitchen floor, he proclaimed, "We need a professional sprinkler guy. And an electrician."

"An electrician? For a sprinkler?"

"For a new timer box. I stuck my screwdriver in there to adjust it and *bam*! Sparks started shooting out all over the place."

"You put a screwdriver in something electrical?" I asked. "You could have burned the house down."

"Relax. Once I figured out which way to point the fire extinguisher, everything was fine."

As he strode into the bathroom, removing his flame retardant-soaked T-shirt, I returned to my call.

"I'm sorry, Donna. What were you saying?"

"Mike," she said. "Talking about how lucky you are to have him."

"*Lucky* doesn't even begin to describe it," I said. Then I told her I'd be over around eight.

Sitting at Donna's computer a few hours later, she pulled up her picture and profile on the screen. But it wasn't Donna's name at the top of the page.

"Miss Triple D?" I blurted. "Who is that?"

"Me. That's my screen name," she said proudly.

"Miss Triple D?" I said incredulously.

"Gets your attention, doesn't it?" she asked with a cocky grin.

"Uh, yeah. But aren't you exaggerating just a . . . lot?"

"It stands for Divine Doll Donna. Neat, huh?"

"Yeah, neat," I said.

"Check out my bio," Donna told me.

According to her profile, "Miss Triple D" is forty-nine years old, she's single, and she loves museums and Bach.

The Donna I know is fifty-six. She's twice divorced and her museum experience consists of one visit to Madame Tussaud's House of Wax. The only musical "Bach" she's ever listened to was Bachman-Turner Overdrive.

As I continued reading, I became more and more amused at Donna's creativity about her life. I managed to keep quiet . . . but when I saw what she'd listed as her favorite hobby, I laughed out loud.

"What?" she asked.

"Pole dancing?!"

"Yeah," she said.

I howled at the image of my friend Donna, her legs wrapped sensuously around a fire pole with crisp dollar bills packed into her cleavage. But then I saw that she wasn't laughing.

"You're serious?" I asked her.

"I took a class last year," Donna confessed. "I'm pretty good at it, too."

I was speechless.

"I didn't tell you because I thought you'd laugh."

"Me? No." Then we both started laughing.

After I finished reading her profile, she asked if I had any suggestions.

"Just a couple . . . You might want to google 'Bach' . . . and I see you left out anything about being a grandmother."

"Yeah, I thought about that," she said. "You know I adore my grandkids but if I put 'proud grandmother of two,' guys could get the wrong impression. . . . You know like instead of thinking I might enjoy an occasional roll in the hay, I belong to a quilting group instead."

We spent the next couple of hours sorting through the website's available men, trying to find her the perfect guy. In her profile, Donna had stipulated that she was only interested in men 40–50.

We almost went with "Corvette Ken," an engineer from Santa Monica, but he was a classical music buff, and Donna was afraid that "Bach" thing might come back to bite her.

Among the other finalists were "All Night Long," a saxophone player from Hollywood; "Road Warrior," an L.A.P.D. motorcycle cop; and a dentist whose screen name was, believe it or not, "Open Wide 4 Me."

Finally, at seven minutes after ten o'clock, we selected the winner of the "Go-to-a-wedding-with-Donna Sweepstakes": "ForePlay," a forty-six-year-old, divorced golf professional from Orange County. His picture was extremely attractive, and among his interests he listed "ballroom dancing," which was one of Donna's passions.

Donna made her selection and heard from him the very next day. His name was Doug, and he'd love to go to the wedding with her. I talked to her the morning afterward, and she told me they'd had an absolutely fantastic time.

He was a really nice guy, and it didn't hurt that they were the hit of the dance floor.

Doug called her two days later to invite her to dinner, and they began dating regularly . . . and seriously. I asked Donna if Doug still thought she was forty-nine.

"Of course," she said.

"And your grandchildren?"

"All in good time," she said.

Apparently, the fates determined that it was a "good time" when they were on their way to our house for dinner; it would be the first time we'd be meeting Doug. He and Donna had stopped at a market to pick up wine and when they were in the checkout line, Donna heard a young, familiar voice boom out from the soda section.

"Grandma!"

Donna turned in time to see her five-year-old grandson, Adam, racing toward her, arms spread for a big hug.

Forty-nine-year-old pole dancer or not, Donna was—first and foremost—a grandmother. Without giving a thought to Doug, she crouched and wrapped herself around Adam as he rushed into her arms.

"You sure look pretty, Grandma," Adam said.

"And you look handsome yourself," Donna told him. "So tell me, what are you doing in this part of town?"

"I'm sleeping over at my friend Jason's," he explained, pointing to another young boy and his father. Donna waved at them, and then became aware of Doug staring down at her. She stood slowly to begin an uncomfortable introduction, "Doug, this is my . . ."

But before she could finish, Adam said happily. "Hi, Doug!"

"Hey, Adam, whassup?" Doug answered, slapping five with the little one.

Donna later told us at dinner that that was the first time in her life she was truly speechless. Finally, she gathered herself enough to babble, "You two know each other?"

"Yeah," Adam said, then looked to Doug, "Can I tell her?"

Doug smiled and nodded.

"See, I came over to your house to get my soccer ball . . ." Adam told his grandmother.

"Last Saturday night before we left for the movies," Doug said, filling in the blanks. "You were running late, and I was waiting downstairs, remember?"

Donna nodded numbly.

"I rang the doorbell and Doug opened the door," Adam said. "And I said, 'Hi, are you my grandma's new boyfriend?'"

"Oh, really . . ." She turned to Doug. "And what did you say?"

"I don't remember," Doug said with a smile.

"Why didn't you tell Grandma about this, Adam?" Donna asked sweetly.

"Doug said it would be a secret. Then we found my soccer ball and Doug gave me two dollars. He's awesome!"

As Donna gave Doug an accusing smile, she noticed that Adam's friend and his father were getting impatient.

"Nice seeing you, sweetie," she said to Adam, giving him a big kiss. "Have fun tonight."

"Thanks, grandma! Bye, Doug!"

And he ran off with his friend.

"Okay," Donna said. "I'm a grandmother."

Doug smiled. "And a very cute one," he added.

They laughed and he put his arm around her. As they walked to the car, Doug suggested to Donna that if they were going to continue together, they'd have to do it honestly.

"Agreed," Donna said. And they shook on it.

Doug sighed. "So, in the interest of honesty, I have to tell you that I'm really fifty-one," he confessed.

"Really?" Donna said. "What do you know . . . So am I," she said, deciding that some truths are better left unspoken.

"And what about that pole dancing thing?" Doug asked.

"What do you mean? That's true."

"Yeah, right," he scoffed.

"Really. It is," she insisted.

But he still didn't believe her, so later that night, thanks to a basketball standard that she'd always intended to have removed from her back yard, Donna proved it.

TWELVE

"TEACH YOUR (GRAND)CHILDREN WELL . . ."

*W*hen Bill and Marge Hankerson retired, they moved from Buffalo to a beautiful senior community in sunny San Diego. They loved everything about their new environment . . . except that it was so far away from their only grandchild, twelve-year-old Garrett.

So they were thrilled when Garrett's parents allowed him to come out for a visit.

On the drive home from the airport, Garrett—who had never been away from home—talked non-stop about all the places he wanted to see during his stay.

"Disneyland, Sea World . . . But most of all, I want to see the ocean!"

"Then tomorrow, that's what we'll do," Marge said.

"You'll love it," Bill continued. "There are so many beautiful beaches."

"Yeah," said Garrett, referring to the tour book he'd been reading on the plane. "It says here that one of the best places called La Jaw-la."

"Where?" Marge asked, having never heard of such a place.

"La Jawla," Garrett repeated, showing his grandmother his book. "See? L-A- J-O-L-L-A."

Marge laughed. "Oh, no, honey," she said. "That's pronounced La Hoy-a," she explained. Garrett frowned. "What?"

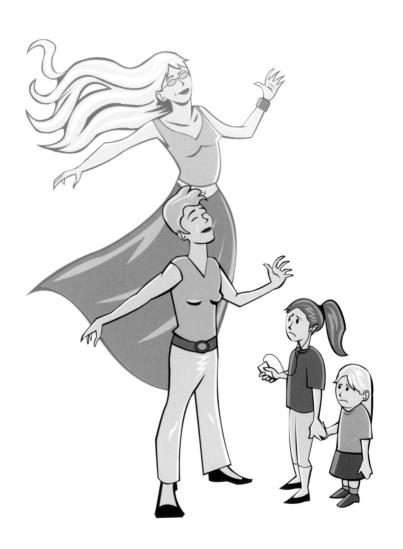

"You see," Marge continued, "because of the Spanish influence out here in California, we pronounce the J's like H's."

"Really?"

"Yep," she said, looking at his tour book. "Like this place," she said, pointing to the name El Cajon, a nearby town.

"El Kay-Jon?" Garret asked, looking at the words.

"No, Gar," Bill said tenderly. "It's pronounced El Ca-hone."

"Remember," Marge reminded him, "in California, we pronounce the J's like H's. Just like in Tijuana, Tujunga, Baja . . ."

Garrett nodded. He understood. Wow, California was a stranger place than he'd heard.

"So Gar," Bill said, "I hear you're doing football camp this summer."

Garrett thought for a moment about what he'd just learned.

"Yep," he said proudly. "Last week of Hune and first week of Huly."

★　★　★　★　★

No matter how many poles grandmas dance on, or rollerblades we ride, or ski hills we conquer, the reality is that our grandchildren will still see us as old . . . regardless of how young we might think we are.

Several years ago, our granddaughter Sydni, then eleven or so, was preparing an oral presentation for school, and, somehow, her subject was Fleetwood Mac's Stevie Nix. When I mentioned that I had once seen Fleetwood Mac in concert, she was amazed.

"You saw Stevie Nicks sing?" she asked.

"Yep," I said, thinking this was definitely earning me some "hip grandma" points. "Wow," Sydni said. "I didn't know she was *that* old." I was glad I didn't mention The Supremes, because if I'd told her I saw Diana Ross, Sydni would have probably thought I was talking about Betsy Ross's sister.

But as the saying goes, "Age brings wisdom." Of course, it also brings sore joints, extra chins, and the need for comfortable walking shoes. But the upside is, because our grandchildren see us as old, they also see us as wise. And while that can be a good thing, wisdom—like most everything that's enjoyable today—comes with a warning: CAUTION: BECAUSE YOUR GRANDCHILDREN SEE YOU AS WISE AND TRUSTWORTHY, THEY WILL OFTEN EXPECT YOU TO REVEAL CERTAIN TRUTHS THAT THEIR PARENTS WON'T.

This rule is particularly important if what you tell them involves either *your* younger days, or those of their parents. For example, let's say your nine-year-old granddaughter says to you, "Nana, mommy told me that when she was my age, she cleaned her room every day and did all her homework as soon as she got home from school."

"Your mother? Room clean? Homework? Are you kidding? When your mother was your age, the cat box was cleaner than her room. And doing homework right after school? I almost had to tie her to the kitchen table so she'd finish it before she went to bed. 'I'll finish it in the morning' she'd say. Then I'd tell her, 'You either finish it now, or you won't be here in the morning.'"

But you don't tell her any of this, because as a grandmother, you don't want to undercut what your child is trying to do as a parent. So what you say to your granddaughter is, "Yep, that's pretty much how your mother was. And she always ate her vegetables, too."

It's important that a grandmother know and accept that their children are the primary teachers for their grandchildren. But every once in awhile, a grandma may find herself called upon to educate a grandchild about some important facet of life.

Consider our friend Carol and her young grandson, Jack, who were on their way to see a movie together. As they waited at a red light, a very, very pregnant woman passed in the crosswalk in front of them.

"Wow, that lady is fat!" said the seven-year-old.

"No, she's not fat," Carol said. "She's pregnant."

"What's that?" Jack asked.

Suddenly, Carol had a grandmother decision to make. If she told her grandson the truth, she might be treading on parental territory. But if she said, "You better ask your parents," Jack might take this to mean that there was something deep, dark, mysterious, and nasty about the process that brought us all to this planet. So which way would Carol go with this one?

"It means she's going to have a baby," Carol finally said.

"But why is she so fat?" Jack asked.

Carol knew she needed to proceed carefully. "Because, honey, she has a baby in her tummy."

Jack looked up at his grandmother as if she'd told him that Santa had just barbecued Rudolph and served him at the elves' annual picnic. "What?" he demanded.

"That's where all babies come from, honey," Carol told him. "From their mommies' tummies."

Jack stared at her for a moment, then, "Even me? Did I come out of my mommy's tummy?

"Yes, honey, you did," Carol said, feeling good about how readily Jack was grasping the concept. She allowed herself to think ahead a few years to when Jack's father would give him "the talk." When it got awkward, Jack could say, "It's okay, Dad; Grandma Carol already explained everything to me."

"Are you sure, Grandma? I really came out of my mom's stomach?"

"I'm sure," she said.

"Wow," the seven-year-old said with a sigh. "Didn't that hurt her mouth?"

As Carol tried to figure out how to respond, the light turned green. She stepped on the gas and said, "Not at all, Jack. Your mom is a very strong woman."

Good luck with that one, Dad.

THE TIMES, THEY ARE A CHANGIN'

Virtually every generation of young mothers has had to deal with *their* mothers looking over their shoulders and offering advice. "Well, *you* can do it however you want . . . it's your baby . . . But here's how *I* did it when you were a girl. . . ." In fact, in the research I've done for this book, I've discovered only one mother who was able to raise her children without instructions from parents before her: her name was Eve something-or-other. Granted, one of her sons had some "brother" issues, but hey, so do the Baldwins.

Even though I was a very young mother, my mom was pretty good about letting me find my own way, except for one thing. . . . and it starts with the letter "P" and ends with "A-C-I-F-I-E-R."

"I don't know why you give her one of those things," she'd say, as if I'd suggested that my baby take a nap holding a live tarantula. "I never needed that when you were a baby."

"There's nothing wrong with a baby sucking its thumb once in awhile," my mom would continue. "It's natural."

Yes, as natural as my bent teeth and two years in orthodontics.

My mom's disdain of the binky was a view held by many mothers of her generation. The reason? They didn't have pacifiers when they were young mothers, so why should we?

But she did admit that she was jealous of a few modern conveniences I had that made mothering easier. These

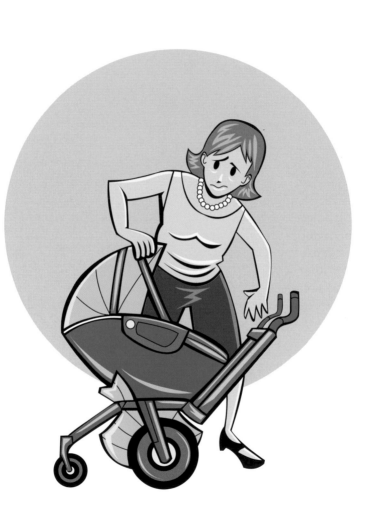

included disposable diapers, Tommee Tippee cups, and *Mister Rogers' Neighborhood*.

And while I may have had it easier than my mom did, I'm learning that mothering can be much more difficult for my daughters' generation than it was for mine. I think there are two factors contributing to this: today's number of working mothers and what I call the "The Business of Babyhood."

WORKING MOMS

There all sorts of reports and statistics regarding the number of mothers in the workplace today, and a detailed analysis of the impact of the trend is better left to sociologists, human behaviorists, and grandmothers living in Boca Raton.

What I *do* know is that every woman who's ever done it without a nanny knows how difficult and exhausting it is to hold a job and be a mom. And even though life was a constant scramble when I did it thirty years ago, there were fewer mothers working, so it was not nearly as difficult to find trustworthy and nurturing daycare as it is today. There were no "waiting lists," no pre-acceptance interviews, and no need to qualify for a home equity loan to pay for it. That so many women have to spend at least half of their salary on child care is appalling. But that's the thing about moms—they'll work as hard as it takes to make sure their kids get what they need—especially health insurance.

I thought about all this recently, when I flashed back thirty years to one of my worst "working mom" days. It was 7:30 one 1973 morning, and—as usual—I was hustling to get my five-year-old daughter to preschool and my two-year-old to day care and still make it to work at a reasonable time. We were just about to leave our apartment when the older one dumped a bowl of cereal on the floor, and I knew that if I left it there all day, I'd need a jackhammer to clean it up when I got home.

After five minutes of nifty mop work, we were at my car out front, where my daughters watched as I unlocked the doors and loaded their stuff into my spiffy 1970 Gremlin. It was then that my beautiful two-year-old decided that, since I'd just put a nice new dress on her, it would be a perfect time to wet her pants. So back into the house we ran, and by the time we pulled away from the curb, I was running thirty minutes behind schedule. But I figured if I drove just a little over the speed limit and hit all the signals, maybe I could make it to work on time. Or close to it.

I was making up a lot of time until the five-year-old looked out the back window and exclaimed, "Mommy, there's a fire engine coming!" Well, it turns out that to a five-year-old, anything with blinking lights looks like a fire engine. What she actually saw was a policeman, and I felt confident that he wasn't pulling me over to tell me how much he liked my Farrah Fawcett hairdo.

Forty-five minutes and a $75 ticket later, I walked into my office, only to find my boss standing by the door, holding a telephone. When he handed me the earpiece, I thought I had a call, and I wondered what it could be now. . . . One of the girls forgot her lunch? The younger one wet her pants again? But when I put the receiver to my ear, what I heard was the recorded voice of the "time lady" reciting the exact time of day, down to the second. My boss smiled sarcastically and walked away. Gee, one of the funniest mid-level incompetents I'd ever worked for.

I was reminded of that incident a few days ago when I was in line at the supermarket behind a young, attractive, well-dressed working mom who had obviously just picked up her four-year-old from daycare on her way home from work. The child was cranky and began a tantrum when his mother refused to buy him one of the sugar-laden candy bars those devil people always place right by the checkout stand.

The little boy's arms and legs tightened, his face grew the color of red that every mother knows will be very soon followed by a scream normally reserved for a Freddy Krueger movie. And sure enough: "Waaaaahhhhh!"

As any experienced mother knows, the child's wailing is the least aggravating component of this scenario. The worst part is when you feel everyone in the entire zip code staring at you and thinking one of two things: 1) "What is that horrible woman doing to that adorable little boy?" or 2) "What a brat! She oughta smack him one!" (Note: These people are usually non-mothers. Or men.)

As the boy continued screeching, a flush of embarrassment came over the poor woman's cheeks. But fortunately, her ordeal would soon be over; her groceries had all been bagged, and as soon as she paid, she could leave the store and give her son a good scolding as soon as she got outside. With her child's shrieking now louder than a group of teenage girls at a Jonas Brothers concert, the mother reached for her purse. But the strap broke and the purse opened up and everything in it—keys, coins, wallet, comb, brush—spilled onto the floor. She stooped to gather her things, and I jumped in to help. We were able to collect everything except for an item that had rolled to the feet of the fifteen-year-old bag boy. He held up an unfamiliar looking tube and chirped to the male checker, "Dude, what is this?"

Without saying a word, the embarrassed mother snatched her tampon holder from him and stuffed it back into her purse.

As she rolled her cart out of the store, I checked my watch. It was nearly 6:30, yet she had still had to go home, unload the groceries, make dinner, do dishes, and get her son to bed. Then she'd fall asleep during the news, and get up and do it all over again tomorrow.

I forget the exact lyrics to that old "M-O-T-H-E-R" song, but if the "H" isn't for "hero," it sure as hell should be.

THE BUSINESS OF BABYHOOD

When I was a young mother, I was appreciative that I had so many more "baby" conveniences available to me than my mother did. Every town had at least one cute little Mom and Pop baby shop named Bonnie's Baby House or Peggy's Playpen, and mothers of that era assumed that these stores carried every possible device a young parent could ever need to raise a healthy, happy, and successful child.

But after a recent trip to a modern baby mega-store, I discovered that all these years, we've apparently been mistaken.

I'm not sure who determined that "variety is the spice of life." Maybe it was the shopkeeper who opened the first variety store, or the writers who created the first variety show, or Liz Taylor. But if the variety of today's baby products were a spice, it would be one of those hot peppers they keep in jars at Mexican restaurants. . . . When something's hot, everyone wants one.

It's both incredible and a bit disheartening to see how today's young parents are being targeted to buy what they're told are absolute "must-haves" for raising a healthy and happy baby.

If you're a grandmother—or about to become one—and haven't yet been to one of these places, here are a few tips to guide you through your first trip. First, if you have a husband who is prone to blurting things like "Holy S#@%!" or "Are you friggin' kidding me?" or "What kind of bozo is gonna spend that much for a $#@&ing high chair?!" then you might want to leave him at home. However, if there's a nearby sports bar with good senior specials, drop him there so you can enjoy two hours of uninterrupted shopping. And if that bar is also a Hooters, you may be good for a three-day weekend.

Upon entering this building the size of an aircraft hangar, you will see a newsstand full of magazines that claim to be chock-full of important, recently-discovered child-rearing tips. These New Age publications have names like *Happy Baby, American Baby*, and just plain *Baby*, who I can only assume is both unhappy and un-American. Then, once babies get older, there's *Child, Parenting, Exceptional Parent, Parent and Child*, and *Family Fun*. Interestingly, there's also a magazine called *Mothering*, but none called *Fathering*. And finally, I spied a publication that touted: *Special Edition: How to Raise a Green Baby*. I understand what "green" means in today's context, but if I'd wanted "green" daughters back when I was a young mom, all I had to do was feed them a regular diet of my Aunt Margie's "chicken surprise."

After leaving the publications section, you will likely find yourself in what I can only describe as the Great Wall of Nipples. These protuberances come in all shapes and sizes, and each is available in something called Level 1 through 4. I admit that I'm not an expert on the subject of nipples.

In high school, I hid my eyes in the girls' locker room, and I was never much for reading National Geographic. But three full aisles of them? I recalled that when I was in the nipple phase, I didn't have to make a choice—there was only one kind. I wondered how new mothers could possibly wade through all the marketing and choose the right nipple for their babies. Do they go to professional nipple makers and have them make latex molds of their breasts?

While examining the vast and confusing selection, I found it curious that while every nipple was made of either rubber or latex, all were advertised as "completely natural." It seems that this is false advertising unless, of course, the baby's mother is an offspring of Gumby.

After leaving "feeding aids," you should go to the stroller section, which has changed a lot since I last owned a stroller. In the dictionary, "stroll" is defined as "a leisurely walk often taken in an idle manner." And that perfectly describes what I used to do with my daughters when they were little—We *strolled*, which allowed them the time to be spellbound by the wonder of a passing butterfly, and to pet our neighbor's dog while he stole a soggy animal cracker from their tray, and to laugh uproariously when I'd tilt the stroller onto its back wheels and say "vrooom-vroom" and then perform a wheelie.

But instead of leisurely walks, some of today's strollers look like they were designed for the Indy 500—others have wheels usually only seen at tractor pulls.

Here's an actual description of one model: *Adjustable suspension, 3-position tilt seat, and aluminum chassis built for both rough terrain and speed*. Rough terrain and speed? I wondered if this stroller was designed to take a baby for a walk, or to escape an erupting volcano. And here's the best part . . . the price: $1,200.

There's another piece of equipment in this department that you should take a look at: it's what we used to call a "walker." Remember that thing that was shaped like an upside down space capsule that you'd put your toddler in while you were cooking dinner? He'd start by kicking his legs spasmodically, but would eventually discover that by putting one foot in front of the other, he could get from one place to the next, where he could get into more trouble than where he just was.

Well, today—and I'm not kidding you here—these things are called "mobile activity centers," and they look like walkers on LSD. There's one called the "Garden" activity center, in which a child can sit amid colorful flowers, complete with a plastic butterfly that looks just like the real one he missed yesterday when his father took him out for a 27 mph "stroll." The big difference between an activity center and a walker is that the activity center doesn't allow the child's feet to touch the ground, which pretty much takes the "walk" out of "walker."

Curious, I asked a sales person about this. When I suggested that old-fashioned walkers seemed to do a better job of introducing a child to the concept of self-propulsion, she stared at me as though I'd said, "For *really* white teeth, I suggest brushing with swimming pool acid."

"Ma'am," she said politely (but not really). "Recent studies suggest that children develop better ambulation skills if they can see their feet when they take their first steps."

Oh, my . . .

My head was spinning as I spent the next two hours wandering though the rest of the store where I learned that what we once called playpens are now called "play yards," even though they're primarily used indoors. I grinned as I thought of George Carlin and his riff on mutually exclusive expressions like "military intelligence" and "jumbo shrimp." I think "inside yard" might also qualify.

Driving home, I found myself feeling genuinely sorry for today's young parents. It seems they simply must have whatever it is they're told is essential to be responsible and caring moms and dads.

But that sympathy didn't stop me from coming up with an invention that would surely be a huge seller in today's lucrative baby marketplace. I don't have it all thought out yet, but it involves a toddler wearing mirrored antennae on his head that would enable him to see his rear end. I figured if being able to see their feet helps babies walk better, think what this could do for potty training.

FOURTEEN

WE ARE FAMILY . . .

*B*etween innings of a little league game, the coach removed one of his nine-year-old players from the game and called him aside for a little chat.

"Jimmy," said the coach, "do you understand what cooperation is?"

Jimmy nodded solemnly.

"And," the coach continued, "what it means to be part of a team?"

"Sure, coach," Jimmy said seriously.

"Do you understand that whether we win or lose, what's important is that we do it together . . . as a team?"

"Yeah, coach."

"And you know that when an umpire makes a call that you don't agree with, you shouldn't argue, curse, attack the umpire and call him a blind tub of goo?"

"Yes, coach. Absolutely," Jimmy answered.

"And do you understand that when I take you out of the game for an inning so one of your teammates gets a chance to play, it's not nice to call your coach a butt face?"

"Of course I know that," said Jimmy.

"Good," said the coach. "Now go up into the grandstands and explain all that to your grandmother."

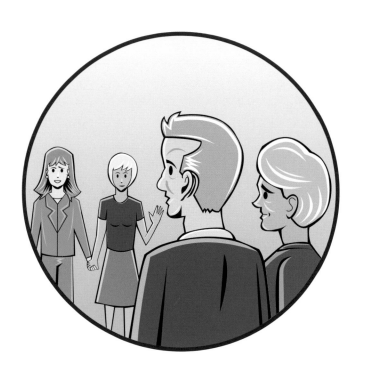

Like the grandmother in that story most grandparents think their grandchild is the cutest and most talented young one on the planet. That's how we're supposed to think; it's in the Grandparents Training Manual. The following story comes from our neighbors, Teri and Jim, who told us about two of their grandparent friends, Chuck and Katrina. As Teri and Jim tell it, Chuck and Katrina are quite possibly the cutest, proudest, and most involved grandparents they know. Chuck and Katrina absolutely adore their vibrant seven-year-old granddaughter, Sara, who is the only child of their only child, Lauren. Whenever they're with Sara—which is often—their eyes dance at the sight of her. Sara is a polite and delightful little girl who is the absolute center of their universe. Chuck and Katrina would never miss one of Sara's soccer or softball games. They sit front row, center, for every one of her school events. Chuck even plays Santa Claus for the Christmas party at little Sara's school. They shudder to think what their lives would be without the joy Sara brings them.

★   ★   ★   ★   ★

There is nothing they wouldn't do for their granddaughter, and they recently hosted Sara's seventh birthday party at their house, complete with clowns, amusements, and pony rides. For her sixth birthday, they took Sara's entire first grade class on a sail around a local harbor. For her fifth birthday, it was Sea World; her fourth, Knott's Berry Farm; her third, LEGOLAND; and on Sara's second birthday, Chuck and Katrina took the entire family to Hawaii for a week.

But on Sara's first birthday, Chuck refused to celebrate. In fact, no matter how much Katrina begged him to reconsider, Chuck would not acknowledge that he even *had* a grandchild. And he hadn't spoken to their own daughter, Lauren, in well over a year.

This was because Lauren, you see, is gay.

Teri and Jim have known Chuck and Katrina since Lauren was a cute, energetic, and smart fifteen-year-old student at a magnet high school here in Los Angeles. She excelled in languages, was a member of the drama society, and headed up the debate team. Lauren's social life was pretty much standard for a teenage girl: movies, parties, boyfriends . . .

Chuck and Katrina were justifiably proud of Lauren, and were over the moon when she graduated from her accelerated high school program with a 4.2 GPA and accepted a scholarship to study pre-law at Harvard.

During Lauren's junior year of college, Teri and Jim were in Boston visiting friends and had set a night aside to take Lauren to dinner. They looked forward to seeing her; Lauren was always fun to be with. And since they hadn't seen her since she left California, they had a lot to catch up on.

"Can I bring my roommate?" Lauren asked Jim when he called to arrange dinner. "She'll pay for herself," she added quickly.

Jim insisted that it would be his treat, and Lauren picked a restaurant near Jim and Teri's hotel.

Teri and Jim arrived a little early, and when Lauren bounded in, they were amazed at the change in her. She had never been a wallflower, but the now twenty-one-year-old Lauren walked into the restaurant with the self-assurance of a cat burglar. As soon as she saw Teri and Jim, she grabbed her roommate by the hand and they ran toward them. Lauren threw her arms around her friends from California and smothered them with kisses.

She then introduced her roommate, Gina, who was every bit as vivacious as Lauren. During dinner, Teri and Jim learned that Gina was a pre-med student from New York City and that she and Lauren had been roommates for a more than year.

"Thirteen months and eight days," Lauren said with a smile.

As the evening went on, Jim and Teri picked up little hints that Lauren and Gina were likely more than roommates to each other. Neither said anything specific, nor did they do anything even close to blatant or overt. It was just the normal things they noticed—how the young women looked at each other, the way they laughed together. Several times, Lauren raved about Gina's intelligence and commitment while Gina begged Teri and Jim for childhood stories about Lauren.

Teri and Jim told us that they'd had so much fun at dinner that they were the last party to leave the restaurant.

After Lauren and Gina hopped into a cab, Teri and Jim walked back to their hotel and talked about how happy Lauren seemed. They wondered if Chuck, who could be very conservative on some issues, knew of Lauren and Gina's relationship. Jim was quite sure Chuck had no idea, and speculated that perhaps Lauren hoped that he and Teri had connected the dots and might broach the subject with her parents.

But Teri and Jim agreed that even though it was no big deal, family business should stay in the family whose business it was.

The next morning their hotel phone rang; it was Chuck calling from California.

"How did your dinner go with Laur?" he wanted to know.

Jim told him dinner was perfect and that he and Teri had met Lauren's roommate.

"Oh, yeah, Gina," he said. "She's a knockout, huh? She's dating some kid she goes to school with. Just like Lauren."

Chuck and Katrina continued to keep Jim and Teri posted on Lauren's life, and Chuck mentioned that when he'd asked Lauren if she was dating anyone, she'd been somewhat evasive. He and Katrina took this to mean that she had a boyfriend she wanted to keep secret for now.

Two years after their visit to Boston, Chuck called to tell them that Lauren had been accepted to Columbia University's law school in New York City.

"And talk about luck," Katrina added. "Her friend Gina? She'll be going to medical school in New York, so they can still be roommates."

Apparently, Lauren hadn't thought the time was yet right to talk to her parents about it. Or was it possible that Jim and Teri had misread the situation?

They got their answer a few years later when Lauren graduated from law school and Chuck, Katrina, Jim, and Teri went to New York for the ceremony. Afterward, they all went out for dinner—Gina included.

Although it was cause for great celebration—Gina had also been accepted as a cardiology resident at Cornell Medical Center New York and Lauren had been heavily recruited by the New York District Attorney's office—Teri and Jim noticed that there was a slight cloud of nervousness during dinner. But Chuck and Katrina seemed oblivious to it.

"So, sweetie," Chuck said to Lauren, "when will you be coming back to California?" This was followed by a quick glance between the two girls.

A short time later, Katrina said to her daughter, "Oh, Lauren, guess who I saw the other day? Jeff Clements!" Then she explained to Gina that Jeff and Lauren had gone to their high school prom together. Then she turned back to Lauren. "He's coming to New York next month, and he wants to have dinner. I gave him your number."

Lauren smiled weakly. Then she turned to Gina, Jim, and Teri. "Could you guys give me a few minutes alone with my folks?"

"Sure," said Gina quickly. "How about a walk?" she suggested to Jim and Teri.

So the three of them left after Teri told Chuck and Katrina that they'd see them back at the hotel.

During a forty-five-minute walk through Central Park, Gina told Jim and Teri what Lauren was telling her parents: that Gina and Lauren were deeply in love and committed to each other. And recently, they'd had an attorney at the firm where Lauren was clerking make it official by drawing up papers declaring them "domestic partners," with nearly all the rights of a legally married couple.

Gina began crying; Jim and Teri hugged her tight and told her how happy they were for them. And they truly meant it; it was clear to them how the young women felt about each other. Gina wiped her eyes, then looked at Teri and Jim with a mischievous smile.

"You knew, didn't you?"

"Pardon?" Jim asked.

"At our dinner in Boston. You could tell, huh?"

Teri and Jim smiled and admitted that they were pretty sure about it way back then.

"All right!" Gina said. "Laur owes me a dinner!"

Gina explained that she thought they knew, but that Lauren didn't. So they'd bet a dinner on it.

"Well, congratulations. Make sure she takes you someplace expensive," Jim said.

"Oh, I will," Gina said. "Because we've got something else to celebrate too."

Then she gave Teri and Jim a bit of news they didn't see coming.

When they got back to their hotel, they heard yelling coming from Chuck and Katrina's room. Actually, Chuck was yelling. Katrina was crying.

Jim knocked. "You guys okay?" he called through the door.

Without an answer, the door flew open. Inside, Chuck was angrily tossing his clothes into his suitcase.

"What's going on?" Teri asked.

Katrina tried to cover. "Oh, really, it's nothing."

"Nothing?" Chuck bellowed. "Our daughter ripping our hearts out is nothing?"

Uh-oh.

Over the next twenty grueling minutes, here's what Jim and Teri were able to put together based on the yelling and crying. . . . Once Lauren and her parents were alone, she told them in no uncertain terms that she wouldn't be moving to California or anywhere until Gina finished her residency. And no, she didn't want to have dinner with Jeff Clements when he came to New York because she was with Gina, whom she loved. This apparently didn't sit at all well with Chuck, who soon blurted the word, "Lesbo."

This enraged Lauren, who said that not only were she and Gina "Lesbos," but it was all legal, to boot.

Then she delivered what was the knockout punch for Chuck: Lauren was pregnant. She and Gina had gone to a sperm bank and selected a donor to fertilize Lauren. And it worked on the first try. She took a home pregnancy test last week, and . . .

That's all that Chuck heard before running from the restaurant, but only after telling Lauren that as far as he was concerned, she could "have as many babies with her dyke friend as she wanted." But he'd have no part of it.

Jim and Teri tried to calm the waters, saying that a lot of gay couples have children these days and . . .

"Are you siding with her?" Chuck demanded.

"Well, no," Jim said. "It's just that Lauren . . ."

"If you want to stay friends with me," Chuck said, looking Jim squarely in the eyes and his jaws clenched, "don't you ever mention her name around me again."

Teri suggested that maybe they should all go down to the lounge and have a drink to cool off, but Chuck had already called for a car to take him and Katrina to the airport.

And within thirty minutes, they were gone.

Eight months later, Jim and Teri received a note from Gina and Lauren announcing the arrival of Sara Joy Weiss-Cowan, who weighed in at 6 pounds, 8 ounces. They enclosed a picture of the newborn and she was absolutely gorgeous. Teri immediately stuck it on her refrigerator, next to the pictures of her own grandchildren.

Then Teri called Katrina, who said that she and Chuck had also received the note and picture, but that Chuck had torn both up as soon as he saw it. Although she and Chuck were heartbroken over the estrangement with their daughter, Chuck—like many men—was able to compartmentalize things and move on with life.

After she hung up with Katrina, Teri removed the picture from the refrigerator and stuck it in a drawer. Chuck and Katrina came over to their house often, and Teri didn't want the picture to be another dagger in their hearts.

Then, about eighteen months later, the Grandparent Gods must have had enough of this foolishness and decided to step in. Dr. Gina Weiss was offered a clinical professorship at the prestigious UCLA Medical Center.

They told no one in California that they were moving to Los Angeles. Then, one beautiful March Saturday morning, with both Chuck and Katrina's cars in the driveway, their doorbell rang.

As he always did, Chuck answered. And before he knew what was happening, Lauren thrust Sara into his arms. "Like it or not, this is your granddaughter. It's time you get to know her." Then she ran off, hopped into a waiting car, and sped away. Gina drove the car around the block and parked just down the street from the house.

After forty agonizing minutes, Lauren once again rang her parents' doorbell. This time, Katrina answered, and as she locked eyes with her daughter, they embraced and wept. It wasn't long before Chuck heard the commotion and came to the door, hugging Sara mightily. He looked at his granddaughter, then at his daughter, and all he could manage was, "Sara's beautiful. She looks just like you."

Well, after a good amount of fence-mending, their family has never been closer. Lauren is a hot-shot defense attorney in Los Angeles and Gina loves everything about UCLA. Late last year, Chuck was barbecuing for what he calls "his girls"—Katrina, Lauren, Gina, and Sara—when he suddenly felt short of breath. Gina saw him perspiring, evaluated the situation, and immediately called 9-1-1.

Two hours later Chuck had an emergency bypass procedure.

Gina did the surgery.

I relate this story not to influence your feelings on same-sex relationships—that is entirely up to you.

But just remember, trying to pick a perfect mate for your son or daughter is like choosing a career when you're eight years old. Childhood dreams often change with maturity. And because grandparents are usually seen as the most "mature" members of the family, it's oftentimes up to us to support our grandchildren's dreams . . . even when their parents may not.

FIFTEEN

BOYS, TOYS, AND OTHER THINGS

"Gaji, why are boys so freakin' weird?"our fourteen-year-old granddaughter Sydni asked recently after reading a text message that was apparently from a young male of the species. I had to tell her the truth: Boys are weird because they were born that way. How else could she explain that while young girls like to play with dolls, young boys like to dismember them? Girls loved coloring with crayons; boys enjoyed sticking them in their nose. Today's little girls want to grow up and be doctors, lawyers, presidents; boys want to grow up and . . . wait a minute, boys don't want to grow up. Never have.

As I looked at her sitting next to me in the car, text messaging so quickly that I thought her cell phone would explode and raise my car insurance, I realized that my first-born granddaughter was leaving a little girl's world of make-believe behind, and was entering a young lady's world of "Ooooo, your daddy's going to have his hands full." Mother Nature had already begun working her magic on Sydni, and I thought back to when I was her age. . . . The only curves I had above the waist were courtesy of a strategically placed pair of my older brother's athletic socks.

I told Syd a story about my free-spirited friend Karly, who took chest enhancement to a new level, when she opted to stuff her bra with water balloons. And it seemed to work

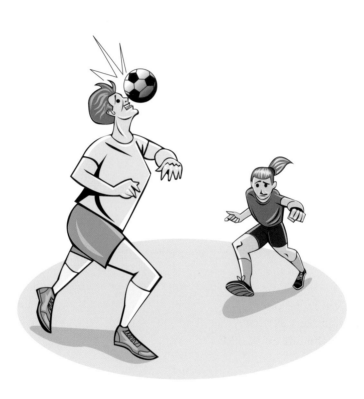

well for her, although she had a slight misadventure when she attended a "boy-girl" thirteenth birthday party. Karly's water balloons were an immediate hit with the guys, and all was going well for her until it came time to play Pin the Tail on the Donkey. The kids circled the blindfolded birthday boy as he tried to stick the donkey with a long hat pin protruding from a paper tail. He was flailing, nowhere near the donkey, when he suddenly stopped and, thinking he was right on target, lurched forward with the pin. Unfortunately for Karly, instead of sticking the donkey's rear end, his pin found one of Karly's water balloons. Bull's-eye! Karly's right breast made like the Wicked Witch of the West and dissolved into a pool of water. As the pre-pubescent boys gaped, my quick-thinking girlfriend was cool as a cucumber.

"My goodness!" Karly exclaimed. "Look how I'm sweating." And before anyone could give it another thought, she hurried into the house to find a bathroom. No more than ten minutes later, she returned completely unaffected, completely dry, and completely stacked. She told me afterwards that she'd dried her blouse with a hair drier and replaced the water balloons with two pieces of wax fruit from an arrangement in the family's dining room.

Pin the tail on *this*, buster!

Sydni and I laughed at this story and as she began to text it to her best friend, I realized that I had just shared a "boobs" story with my granddaughter. Wow, where did the years go?

I'm sure that the time will come that I'll share that benign and innocent story with all my granddaughters. But I've learned that that's as far as any "sex" talks between us should go. That is parents' territory; and they're welcome to it.

Following are a few other helpful lessons I've learned about the grandmother-grandchild relationship that I am happy to pass on.

THANKS, BUT NO THANKS

If you have to *mail* your grandchildren's presents instead of deliver them in person, don't let your feelings be hurt when you send your twelve-year-old granddaughter a pair of stylish jeans and a matching top for her birthday, and don't receive an immediate note of gratitude. What probably will happen is that you'll call her two weeks later to see if she received the package, and all you'll get is a "Yeah, grandma, thanks. They're cool." Your first instinct will be to admonish your daughter, telling her that it's a mother's job to see that her children write thank-you notes. But before you do, I suggest you think back to when your daughter was a little girl and got presents from *your* mother. "Okay," you told her, "tomorrow morning, we are going to write grandma a thank you note." But in the morning, she woke up with a fever and couldn't go to school, and you got called in to work even though it was supposed to be your day off, so you got your neighbor to watch her for the day, and then when you got home, your daughter's fever was gone, but you felt yourself coming down with something, so you forced yourself to stay awake until she fell asleep, then you went to bed and woke up the next morning feeling like you had malaria, even though you had no idea what malaria was, or felt like. But you had to pull yourself out of bed to get her breakfast, make her lunch, and take her to school. Then you came home and fell into bed with a fine case of the chills, and just when you were about to fall asleep, the cable guy arrived to disconnect because you forgot to pay your bill. And . . . and . . . and . . .

And the note to your mother never got written.

Sure, it would be wonderful to receive a thank-you note from your grandchildren every time you sent a present. But then, a lot of things would be wonderful . . . like your husband learning how to work a vacuum in the house as well as he does in his car, like your dog not shedding, and like your sister staying in a relationship for more than two and a half years.

ROAD T(R)IPS

Like many grandparents, we hadn't done any extended travel with young children for awhile, so when we went to Hawaii with our three grandchildren and their parents, it took some re-acclimating.

Before we even got on the plane, we learned a clever tip while sitting in the terminal and waiting to board our flight. Because regulations require that we be at the airport so much earlier these days, it means that parents have even more time to keep their eyes on their antsy children who want scurry into gift shops and kiosks that sell $7 cups of coffee. Ron and Dionn's antennae went up each time one the girls got lost in the crowd, but the young parents sitting next to us didn't seem to have this concern about their children. This is because they had their three young sons, ages ten, seven, and five dressed in identical, God-awful, red and white striped shirts. I asked them about this and they explained that whenever they travel, they make their boys wear their "airport shirts" so they can be spotted immediately, unless, of course, the airport is filled with barber shop quartets. When Mike suggested to Dionn that this might be a good idea for our granddaughters, she politely explained that girls are a bit different, and the last time she dressed Sydni and Samantha alike, they locked themselves in their rooms and demanded to be put up for adoption.

We also learned on that vacation that parents today have to travel with a lot more kiddie gear than we did. With car seats, toy bags, electronic gadgets, a month's worth of clothes for a one-week stay, they had more luggage than a Madonna tour. So since there were seven of us, we decided to be smart and rent a huge, nine-passenger van with an oversized luggage rack. Then we rented a mid-size so Mike and I could get to the hotel, too.

When we spent an entire day touring in the van, Mike and I were reminded that when girls of a certain age— normally eight to sixteen—bicker, the word "no" contains two syllables.

"Give me the iPod," said the eight-year-old to the eleven-year-old.

"No-uh!" was her response, sounding like she was talking about the guy who built the ark.

But touring with our three young grandchildren was great, and there was one unexpected bonus: For once, it wasn't just us requesting bathroom stops.

AND BABY MAKES THREE ALREADY!

Many of my friends are primed to be grandmothers, but their married children have yet to deliver the goods. My friends have nudged, prodded, and done more begging than Heidi Fleiss at an Elks Club picnic.

Because so many of them seem to have this problem, I've come up with a little cattle prod of a solution they might want to try.

Next time your married-without-a-child child calls for a chat, tell him you'd love to talk, but you can't right now, because you and your husband are on your way to your attorney's office to make some changes to your will. Then tell him that you're going to name him as executor because you know that he'll carry out your last wishes to the letter.

"You can count on me," he'll say soberly. Then he'll ask nonchalantly, "Is that all you're changing?"

Now you've got him right where you want him.

"Yeah, that's pretty much it," you tell him. "Except that we're leaving 95 percent of the estate to our grandchildren."

"But we don't have kids yet, Mom," he'll remind you.

"Oh, that's right," you say. "Well, then it all goes to the cat."

It's a good bet there will be a grandchild in the works within the year. If not, ask your son if he knows where you could take skydiving lessons.

CALL IN THE CHOPPERS

We've already talked about how young parents like to leave detailed lists when a grandmother babysits. But for some parents, apparently a list is not enough, and they like to talk a grandmother through tasks she's been performing for years.

This comes from our friend Sharon, whose son Brad is a new, first-time father.

"Okay, good," Brad said to Sharon, looking over her shoulder as she removed a soiled diaper from her three-week-old granddaughter. "Next, you have to clean her bottom," Brad said, as though explaining some revolutionary concept. Then he removed a baby wipe from a "warmer" and handed it to her. "We've started keeping them in a warmer, because cleaning her with a cold one could be a shock to her."

"Oh," Sharon said with a sigh. "Where did you use to keep her diapers . . . in dry ice?"

Brad didn't laugh as he continued his instruction. "And make sure you rub her gently. Too hard and she could get a rash," he continued, speaking as though he were the reincarnation of Dr. Benjamin Spock.

These instructions continued throughout the diaper-changing process and only ended when she placed the baby in her crib for a nap.

Sharon says that they're like that every time she's with her granddaughter.

"It bugs me, the way they hover over me," she complains. "They're like helicopter parents."

That Christmas, she gave her son and his wife a gag gift. She pasted small pictures of them on the side of a plastic army helicopter.

They didn't get it.

A CAUTIONARY TALE

I've heard a number of brand-new grandmothers say, "Having a grandchild makes me feel young again." From experience, I know how they feel . . . holding a new baby, changing a new baby, bathing a new baby, enjoying that new baby smell. What these brand new grandmas seem to forget is that new babies become old babies, and old babies become two-year-olds, and two-year-olds can move faster than a grandma can. Then, before you know it, they become five-year-olds who say things like, "Can you pick me up, Grandma, and carry me back to the car?" (which is parked on the third floor of the mall parking lot).

And before long, five-year-olds become eight-year-olds who say, "Can you play soccer with me, Grandma? I won't kick it hard. Promise." You know your granddaughter is very athletic for her age, but you were pretty good at sports when you were a girl, so you figure, "What the heck. What's it gonna hurt?" You find out soon enough when you remove the ice pack from your nose and finish repairing your glasses. It's then that you realize maybe you're not as young as that darling little baby made you feel.

But because you love and enjoy your grandkids so much, there's no way you'll stop playing with them. However, you will have to make slight concessions to your "maturity," and limit your activities to occasional ski trips and things like Uno and Crazy Eights.

But don't be discouraged; that's the nature of things. Everyone knows that you can still kick up your heels. But like a lot of us, just not as high.

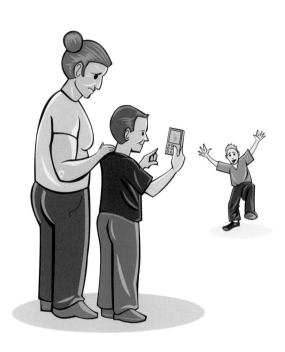

SIXTEEN

IF WISHES WERE KINGS ... OR QUEENS

Here I am at sixty years old. I've been a happy and proud grandmother for nearly fifteen years, and I hope and pray that I have at least another fifteen ahead of me, because this is truly a wonderful time of my life.

But as we get older, we become acutely aware that we don't come with warranties. Some of us get 100,000 miles, others get a quick spin around the block. So before a tree falls on me, or lightning strikes me, or I get abducted by aliens who look the way Brad Pitt looked at the beginning of *Benjamin Button*, I'd like to pass on some hopes and thoughts to our grandchildren. And to yours, if you'd like.

I hope your most recent kiss matches the thrill of your first.

I hope you always dance like no one's watching.

I hope you're never embarrassed to wear a funny hat.

I hope you play your trumpet with Gabriel's certainty and Satchmo's joy.

I hope you can always get in our house when we're not here. (Hint: There's a key hidden on the back porch in the ceramic porcupine. Ssshhhh!)

I hope you embrace travel. In discovering other people, you often discover yourself.

I hope your driving instructor has a sense of humor.

I hope you don't rely on Cliff's Notes.

I hope your glass slippers always fit.

I hope you see education as a gift, not a chore.

I hope you have time to come down and help us clean our garage . . . again.

I hope you remove your earphones often enough to hear laughter. And weeping.

I hope for a cure for cystic fibrosis, so Alex can be a grandma, too.

I hope you give foreign films another chance . . . even ones with birds.

I hope that once a month, you eat something you've never tried before.

I hope you can teach Buh-Buh how to take pictures with his cell phone.

I hope when you encounter a wall between dreams and reality, you knock it down.

I hope you find someone who inspires you.

I hope you always vote.

I hope you never have to see another Rocky *sequel.*

I hope you get to see Tony Bennett in concert when he's 103.

I hope you learn a second language . . . then a third, and a fourth.

I hope you experience the joy of volunteerism.

I hope you always enjoy warm pumpkin pie with mounds of whipped cream.

I hope we can go to Disneyland together again. (But this time, you have to push us through Fantasyland in strollers.)

I hope you set foot on the moon. If not, Italy will do.

I hope poets and songwriters always amaze you.

I hope you learn to fix your own car and put on your own snow chains.

I hope you'll buy a meal for someone who hungers. And not brag to anyone about it.

I hope you experience the joy of Christmas every day.

I hope your heart melts when you hear a baby laugh.

I hope the letters "SUV" will return to just being part of the alphabet for you.

I hope when you light candles to guide your way, you will recognize me as one of them.

I hope when all your friends offer advice, you only listen to the one who has a dog.

I hope if you ever have a crisis of faith, you talk to someone who's had one, too.

I hope that when you do your laundry, you have enough quarters and dimes.

I hope than when you get pulled over for speeding, a certain CHP officer has retired.

I hope that instead of getting paid by the hour, you get paid by the thought.

I hope that if people march to a different drummer, you hold the drumsticks.

I hope that my mother can see how spectacular you are.

I hope that when you fall asleep at night, goodness is your pillow.

I hope that when all else fails, your family won't.

I hope you will read many wonderful things.

And finally . . .

I hope you will experience the burning love I have for you.

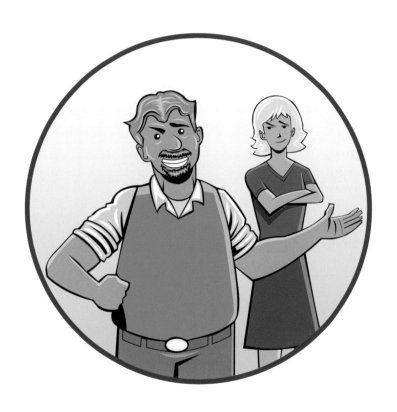

AFTERWORD
by Mike Milligan

I would like to take a few minutes to brag about Jill. And because I have attained the exalted rank of Grandfather, you are required to do what you usually do when an older man tells a story: Be polite and pretend to listen. Then, when I am finished, you can immediately forget every word. Just like I probably will.

I must start by telling you what a fantastic grandmother Jill is. Her grandchildren adore her; they think she is beautiful, funny, smart and "totally rad" to be around. They are very perceptive.

In addition to the above qualities, Jill is amazingly patient and giving. In her almost fifteen years of grandmotherhood, I have never once seen her lose her patience with any of our grandchildren, no matter how cranky or demanding they can be at times. Even more incredibly, she hardly ever loses her patience with *me* when I say or do something foolish, an occurrence that happens almost weekly—okay, daily. But who died and made you the shenanigans police?

For the past fifteen years, I have watched in admiration as Jill handles every job requirement of grandmotherhood with ease and competence. She has never, ever, forgotten a grandchild's birthday, school play, or recital. Perhaps I find this so admirable because I still often forget what day the big noisy truck comes to pick up our trash. In observing Jill and her other devoted grandmother friends, I have come to the sobering conclusion that when it comes to grand-parenthood, grand*mothers* carry the ball for all of us, while grand*fathers* try to recall where they left their helmets. Jill is the Sun around which our grandchildren revolve. I, on the other hand, am nothing more than the Pluto . . . or perhaps Goofy. As I have said many times before when quick and incisive grandparent action was needed: When the chips are down, grandmothers know exactly what to do. When the chips are down for grand*fathers*, we just shuffle out to the kitchen and search for more chips.

Think of grandmothers as the stars of their families; grandfathers are just their sidekicks. We are Sonny to their Cher, Abbott to their Costello, Ed McMahon to their Johnny, the Pips to their Gladys Knight. Like an old reliable piece of sturdy luggage, grandfathers are just along for the journey. Our grandmother-wives can drag us wherever they choose, and we gladly go along because we know that they will take care of everything and all we have to do is provide a well-padded lap for our grandkids to sit, an occasional joke, and a healthy supply of gold cards.

What's more, grandfathers reap the benefits of grandmothers' hard work. For example, we receive and gladly accept huge hugs and kisses from our grandkids for gifts that come from "Grandma and Grandpa," even though we're more surprised at what's inside than they are. Also, we have an entire new audience for the stories that have caused old friends to move to another state rather than be forced to sit through them again. And best of all, when we visit the grandkids, we always get the most comfortable bed.

Grandmothers seem to have the talent for saying just the right thing at the right time; they are much better than grandfathers when it comes to teaching our grandchildren important life lessons . . . except for maybe how to hit a ball with any kind of stick. At least until Annika Sorentam becomes a grandmother.

And Jill is a master of all these talents and more. But as wonderful as she is, I've learned that she can sometimes fall into flurries of gross exaggeration. That's why I believe it's my duty to set the record straight about a few less-than-flattering things she wrote about me in the book you've just read. And remember, I am not doing this for myself—I am doing it for grandfathers everywhere.

For starters, my tool collection does *not* consist of only a "large screwdriver and a pair of pliers." I also have a small power saw I bought at an estate sale. I've only used it once, when I tried to install a doggie door at our house. It wasn't an entirely successful venture, but the vet was correct when she assured us that our mutt's tail would eventually heal on its own. Our loyal dog has pretty much forgiven me for that mishap, although she still runs for cover whenever I switch on my electric shaver.

Next, I do not have any Cruex in my medicine cabinet. That was just a cheap joke. I haven't needed an anti-fungal since I stopped playing in that pick-up game at the YMCA.

And when it comes to what Jill describes as my "ample, red, Irish nose" I must take exception. Yes, it is red, and I am of Irish descent . . . but "ample?" Granted, my schnozz might be a little larger than normal. And yes, over the years I've been told I resemble both W.C. Fields and Karl Malden. But no one's ever called me "Rudolph!" And if my blower is so humongous, how is it that I have a moustache? Isn't it impossible to grow anything in the shade?

I hope all this will correct the record and any misimpressions you might have of me.

But in spite of these injustices, I thank Jill for allowing me to help out with this book. We worked surprisingly well together, and on the few occasions when there was a disagreement about the material, we handled it like most mature, long-time couples settle disputes: I quit arguing and did exactly what Jill told me to do. And because of this, I've learned that in our house—particularly when it comes to the grandkids, it's absolutely true: "Grandma Rules."

ACKNOWLEDGMENTS

To Daniel Lazar at The Writers House and Mark Weinstein of Skyhorse Publishing, thanks for the encouragement and opportunity. And I send snow shovels full of appreciation to Lilly Golden, for her splendid editing and re-structuring advice. And to Adam Wallenta for his marvelous illustrations.

Of course, were it not for my precious and gregarious granddaughters Sydni, Samantha, Alexandra, and Claire, who bring so much sunshine and fun into my life, there would be no *Grandma Rules.* So thanks, love, and kisses to you, as well as to my amazing daughters, Dionn and Mischon, who have inspired and encouraged me all my life. And to my outstanding sons-in-law, Ron and Kevin. . . . You're the best.

Huge hugs and kisses to Rochelle, McKenna, Denise R., Zippy and Denise, Paul and Norma, Carmen and Sebastian, Bill and Margrethe, and my good "frin" Karley, who, along with all my other wonderful friends—grandmothers or otherwise—have provided their unflagging support and numerous stories.

A very special tribute to my late sister and brother-in-law, Pat and Larry, who were always, always there for me.

And to my husband. . . . You'll get yours later.

Jill Milligan is an actress and comedian who lives in West Hills, California, which is a tortuous five-hour drive from her four grandchildren. She would like to thank every gas station and burger joint along CA Route 99 for the food, coffee, and bathroom facilities. This is her first book.

Michael Milligan has been writing television comedies for more than thirty years, with credits including *The Jeffersons, Chico and the Man, Good Times, Dear John,* and *All in the Family.* He is also the author of *Grandpa Rules* from Skyhorse Publishing and is a humor writer for the website, *Grandparents.com.*